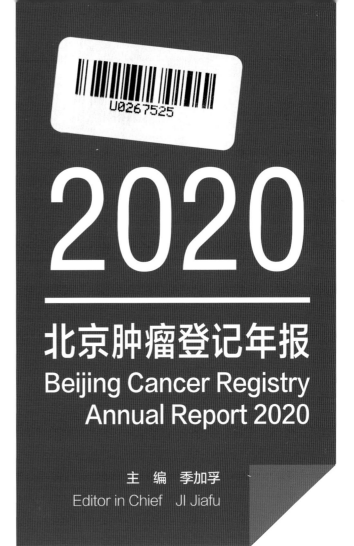

2020

北京肿瘤登记年报
Beijing Cancer Registry
Annual Report 2020

主　编　季加孚

Editor in Chief　JI Jiafu

北京大学医学出版社

2020 BEIJING ZHONGLIU DENGJI NIANBAO

图书在版编目（CIP）数据

2020 北京肿瘤登记年报 / 季加孚主编.—北京：
北京大学医学出版社，2021.4
ISBN 978-7-5659-2339-5

Ⅰ.① 2… Ⅱ.①季… Ⅲ.①肿瘤－卫生统计－北京
－ 2020 －年报 Ⅳ.① R73-54

中国版本图书馆 CIP 数据核字 (2020) 第 247756 号

审图号：京 S（2021）026 号

2020 北京肿瘤登记年报

主　　编：季加孚
出版发行：北京大学医学出版社
地　　址：（100191）北京市海淀区学院路 38 号　北京大学医学部院内
电　　话：发行部　010-82802230；图书邮购　010-82802495
网　　址：http://www.pumpress.com.cn
E - mail：booksale@bjmu.edu.cn
印　　刷：北京信彩瑞禾印刷厂
经　　销：新华书店
策划编辑：董采萱
责任编辑：刘　燕　董采萱　　责任校对：靳新强　　责任印制：李　啸
开　　本：889 mm×1194 mm　1/16　　印张：16.25　　字数：330 千字
版　　次：2021 年 4 月第 1 版 2021 年 4 月第 1 次印刷
书　　号：ISBN 978-7-5659-2339-5
定　　价：180.00 元

版权所有，违者必究
（凡属质量问题请与本社发行部联系退换）

编委会
Editorial Board

主　编
季加孚

副主编
杜　红　黄若刚　王　宁　刘　硕

专家委员会（以姓氏笔画为序）
刘　峰　孙喜斌　杜灵彬　宋冰冰
张思维　郑荣寿　贺宇彤　魏文强

编　委（以姓氏笔画为序）
王　宁　韦再华　刘　硕　刘　晶
杜　红　李　刚　李　俊　李晴雨
李慧超　杨　雷　张　希　张　倩
季加孚　郭默宁　黄若刚　程杨杨
路　凤

Editor in Chief
JI Jiafu

Associate editors
DU Hong HUANG Ruogang WANG Ning LIU Shuo

Committee of experts
LIU Feng SUN Xibin DU Lingbin SONG Bingbing
ZHANG Siwei ZHENG Rongshou HE Yutong WEI Wenqiang

Editorial Board
WANG Ning WEI Zaihua LIU Shuo LIU Jing
DU Hong LI Gang LI JUN LI Qingyu
LI Huichao YANG Lei ZHANG Xi ZHANG Qian
JI Jiafu GUO Moning HUANG Ruogang CHENG Yangyang
LU Feng

前言
Foreword

恶性肿瘤是严重威胁居民生命和健康的一大类疾病，多年来一直是北京市居民的主要死亡原因，且发病呈现逐年上升趋势。肿瘤登记是定期收集某地人群恶性肿瘤发病、死亡和生存数据的系统性工作，是制定肿瘤防治政策、评价防控效果及开展相关研究的基础性疾病监测工作。在北京市卫生健康委员会发布的关于贯彻落实《健康中国行动——癌症防治实施方案（2019—2022年）》有关工作的通知中明确指出要"强化肿瘤登记报告工作，提高报告效率及质量"。

肿瘤登记工作的标志性成果之一就是每年及时向政府和社会发布肿瘤登记监测数据。近年来，北京市肿瘤登记监测数据不仅被国际癌症研究署和国际肿瘤登记协会《五大洲癌症发病率》收录出版，标志着北京市肿瘤登记数据达到国际水平，而且自2010年起由北京市政府通过《北京市卫生与人群健康状况报告》向社会公布，标志着政府对人民健康和肿瘤防治工作的重视。为了提供更丰富详尽的科研监测数据，此次首次出版"北京肿瘤登记年报"。本年报汇总了2017年北京市恶性肿瘤监测数据。截止到2020年6月30日，北京市肿瘤防治研究办公室收到来自全市168家二级及以上医疗机构报送的2017年肿瘤登记数据。此次年报对23种恶性肿瘤及所有恶性肿瘤合计的发病和死亡数据进行了详细的分析，并分地区、年龄和性别比较了恶性肿瘤的分布差异。

《2020北京肿瘤登记年报》的顺利出版，得到了国家癌症中心/全国肿瘤登记中心、北京市卫生健康委员会疾病预防控制处、北京市疾病预防控制中心、北京市卫生健康委员会信息中心和北京大学肿瘤医院的大力支持，凝结着全市近200家医疗机构工作人员的辛苦付出和10余位编写、校审人员的辛勤劳动。北京市肿瘤登记年报的出版发行得益于所有工作人员的支持和付出，在此表示衷心的感谢！

北京市肿瘤防治研究办公室　主任
北京大学肿瘤医院　院长
北京市肿瘤防治研究所　所长
2020年10月

Cancer is a group of numerous distinct disease that intimidates mankind's life and health seriously and has been the leading cause of deaths in Beijing for many years. The incidence of cancer in Beijing also increased gradually in the last few decades. Cancer registration is a systematic work that collects cancer incidence, mortality and survival data for a specific population at regular intervals. Cancer registration is a basic surveillance work which plays an important role for formulating cancer prevention policies, evaluating the impact of cancer prevention and control, and supplying basic evidence for related research. In the Notice on implementing *Healthy China Action- Action plan for Cancer Prevention and Control (2019-2022)* issued by Beijing Municipal Health Commission emphasized that strengthening cancer registry and improving efficacy and quality of data submission.

One prominent achievement of cancer registration in Beijing is to release Beijing cancer surveillance data to public. In recent years the cancer surveillance data in Beijing has been accepted by *Cancer Incidence in Five Continents* published by the International Agency for Research on Cancer (IARC) and International Association of Cancer Registries (IACR) which marked the quality of data in Beijing reached the international level. And the cancer surveillance data were issued to public through the *Health and Population Health Report of Beijing* by the Municipal Government of Beijing since 2010, which indicates that the government attaches great importance to people's health and cancer prevention and control. In order to provide more detailed scientific surveillance data, this is the first time to publish *Beijing Cancer Registry Annual Report*. In this report, cancer incidence and mortality data in Beijing of 2017 were reported. Cancer surveillance data from 168 hospitals in Beijing in 2017 were submitted by Jun. 30, 2020. The report was summarized data of the incidence and mortality for cancer combined and 23 cancer sites in 2017 and was calculated in strata by areas, age and sex.

National Cancer Center & National Central Cancer Registry, Division of Disease Prevention and Control of the Beijing Municipal Health Commission, Beijing Center for Diseases Prevention and Control, Beijing Municipal Health Commission Information Center and Peking University Cancer Hospital provided sustainable support in publication of the *Beijing Cancer Registry Annual Report 2020*. And it also embodies the hard work of staffs from nearly 200 medical institutions and more than ten authors and editors.

I acknowledge the support and dedication of all the staffs who contributed to this publication.

Jiafu Ji

Director of Beijing Office for Cancer Prevention and Control

President of Peking University Cancer Hospital

President of Beijing Institute for Cancer Research

October, 2020

目录

Contents

1 概述
Introduction

1.1 北京市肿瘤登记处概况

北京市肿瘤登记处始建于 1977 年，2010 年归入北京市肿瘤防治研究办公室，隶属于北京市卫生健康委员会疾病预防控制处管理，挂靠在北京大学肿瘤医院和北京市肿瘤防治研究所。目前，登记处有 4 名专职工作人员和 4 名兼职人员，其中博士 3 人，硕士 5 人。

北京市面积为16 410平方公里，位于北纬39°56′，东经116°20′，属于暖温带半湿润半干旱季风气候，年平均降水量为450~750 mm，年平均相对湿度为50%。北京市肿瘤登记处收集的发病和死亡数据覆盖全市16个区的1 361万人口，其中95.9%是汉族，少数民族只占4.1%。

北京是中华人民共和国的首都，也是政治、经济、文化中心，医疗技术水平国内领先，医疗设备完善。北京市卫生健康委员会管辖的 188 家二级及以上医疗机构中，168 家报告肿瘤病例（其中肿瘤专科医院 5 所），其余医院不收治肿瘤患者。

北京市肿瘤登记处通过"北京市卫生综合统计信息平台"收集各医院上报的肿瘤发病和死亡数据。北京市肿瘤死亡信息由北京市疾病预防控

1.1 Brief introduction of Beijing Cancer Registry

The Beijing Cancer Registry (BCR) was founded in 1977 and was merged into the Beijing Office for Cancer Prevention and Control, which is affiliated to the Division of Disease Prevention and Control of the Beijing Municipal Health Commission, in 2010. It also belongs to Peking University Cancer Hospital and the Beijing Institute for Cancer Research. At present, there are four full-time and four part-time employees working with the registry (3 have Ph.D. degrees and 5 have Master degrees).

Beijing is located at the latitude of 39° 56′ N, and the longitude of 116° 20′ E, covering 16,410 square kilometers. It has the typical temperate continental monsoon climate. The average annual precipitation is about 450-750 mm, with the relative humidity 50%. The BCR covers the 16 administrative districts of Beijing, with about 13.61 million inhabitants, 95.9% of whom are Han Chinese and 4.1% from ethnic minority groups.

Beijing, the capital and the political, economic and cultural center of China, boasts the top-notch healthcare facilities equipped with cutting-edge technologies of the country. Among the 188 secondary and tertiary hospitals under the supervision of the Beijing Municipal Health Commission, 168 hospitals have reported cancer case information to the BCR in 2017, including 5 cancer hospitals. The other hospitals that do not treat and report cancer patients were not included into the surveillance.

The BCR collects cancer incidence and mortality data from the "Beijing Health-care Information Statistical Platform" provided by the Beijing Municipal Health Commission. The mortality data are derived from the vital statistics department of the Beijing

制中心的生命统计部门提供，人口资料由北京市公安局提供。

1.2 北京市肿瘤登记体系建设及发展历史

　　肿瘤登记是定期收集某地人群癌症数据的系统性工作，收集的信息包括癌症患者个人信息、诊断信息、治疗信息、随访信息和当地人口资料。肿瘤登记是制定癌症防控政策、评价癌症防控效果及开展相关研究的基础性疾病监测工作。

　　北京市自 1977 年根据《关于建立北京市恶性肿瘤登记报告制度及进行死亡回顾调查的通知》[（76）京卫科学第 191 号] 文件要求，开展以人群为基础的肿瘤登记工作以来，最初采用城区（东城、西城、崇文、宣武、朝阳、海淀、丰台、石景山）医院手工填写报告卡的方式报告首诊病例。20 世纪 90 年代逐步覆盖全市 16 区，并以北京市生命统计部门提供的死亡资料作为发病漏报和死亡结局的补充。2004 年根据《关于加强和落实北京市肿瘤登记报告工作的通知》（京卫办字 [2004]39 号文件），开始通过"北京市卫生综合统计信息平台"的肿瘤登记模块，每月采集全市二级及以上医疗机构的出院病案首页信息，收集癌症患者信息，实现了全市网络直报，减少了漏报率，提高了时效性。

　　2009 年北京市开展覆盖全市的病案核查工作，逐步提高形态学确诊（morphological verification, MV）比例，降低部位不明（other or unspecified sites，O&U）比例和仅有死亡医学证明书（death certificate only，DCO）的比例。2010 年，为了提高生存率的准确性，北京市针对城区的肿瘤现患

1.2 Development history of the cancer registration system in Beijing

Center for Diseases Prevention and Control, and the population data are provided by the Beijing Municipal Public Security Bureau.

Cancer registration is a systematic work that collects cancer data for a specific population at regular intervals. The information being collected includes the demographic, diagnosis, treatment, follow-up and the population data. Cancer registration is a basic surveillance work which plays an important role for formulating cancer prevention policies, evaluating the impact of cancer prevention and control, and supplying basic evidence for related research.

The BCR was founded according to the administrative document of *Establishing Beijing Cancer Registration and Conducting Retrospective Investigation on Death.* The BCR has been collecting population-based cancer information using the manually filled report cards since 1977. The surveillance covered 8 urban districts: Dongcheng, Xicheng, Chongwen, Xuanwu, Chaoyang, Haidian, Fengtai and Shijingshan. In the 1990s, the coverage of the surveillance was gradually expanded, covering all the 16 districts of the city, and supplementary information—the death certificate information from the vital statistics department of the Beijing Centers for Diseases Prevention and Control, was used as a source for missed reporting of cases and the mortality data. According to the administrative document of *Strengthening Data Reporting and Application of Beijing Cancer Registration,* since 2004, we have been using the cancer registration system, a module of the "Beijing Health-care Information Statistical Platform", to collect the patient information monthly from the profile information of the medical records of patients discharged from secondary or tertiary hospitals in Beijing. This made direct online reporting possible, reducing the rate of underreporting and improving the timeliness of data reporting.

In 2009, the BCR re-abstracted the medical record of all related facilities in Beijing to raise the proportion of morphological verified cases (MV%), to reduce the proportion of "other and unspecified cases" (O&U%) and the proportion of cancer cases recognized by death certificate only (DCO%). In order to improve the quality

患者开展主动随访工作，并延续至今。

1.3 年报统计数据

1.3.1 年报数据收集范围

本年报数据收集截止时间为 2020 年 6 月 30 日，数据上报时间范围为 2017 年 1 月 1 日至 2017 年 12 月 31 日。上报医院共计 168 家北京市二级及以上医疗机构。ICD-10 编码收集范围为 C00-97、D00-09、D32-33、D42-43、D45-47，经过核查病历剔除良性肿瘤和原位癌，年报 ICD-10 编码统计范围为 C00-97 和 D45-47。人口数据采用 2017 年年中人口数据，覆盖北京市 16 区户籍人口 13 610 288 人（男性 6 791 497 人，女性 6 818 791 人）。其中城区 6 个（东城、西城、朝阳、海淀、丰台、石景山，原崇文和宣武于 2010 年分别并入东城和西城），覆盖人口 8 440 225 人，占 62.01%；郊区 10 个（门头沟、房山、通州、顺义、昌平、大兴、怀柔、平谷、密云、延庆），覆盖人口 5 170 063 人，占 37.99%。

1.3.2 年报主要统计内容

本年报汇总了 2017 年北京市 16 个区户籍人口癌症的发病、死亡及人口数据。详细描述了北京市肿瘤登记处数据的质量控制指标结果，如 MV%、M/I、DCO%、OU% 等。详细报道了合计癌症和 23 种癌症的发病与死亡数据，指标包括：发病率，死亡率，中国人口标化率（2000 年中国人口构成），世界人口标化率（Segi 世界人口构成），累积率，分城郊、年龄组、性别的发病率及死亡率等。部分癌种按亚部位和组织学分型进行了细节描述。

（撰稿 王宁，校稿 杨雷）

of the data for survival analysis, the BCR has been following up cancer patients who are still alive in the urban areas of Beijing since 2010.

1.3 Data specification in this annual report

1.3.1 Data collection scope

Medical records of newly diagnosed cancer patients and deaths from all the 168 hospitals between Jan.1, 2017 and Dec. 31, 2017 were reported to the BCR by Jun. 30, 2020. According to the International Classification of Diseases 10th Revision (ICD-10), the cases with the codes of C00-97, D32-33, D42-43, D45-D47 were included into the BCR surveillance system, but only the cases with the codes of C00-97 and D45-D47 were included into analysis in this annual report after excluding the benign tumors recognized through medical record verification. The Beijing population in the middle of 2017 was used for incidence and mortality calculation in this annual report. At that time, there were 13,610,288 permanent residents in Beijing (6,791,497 males, 6,818,791 females, respectively), with 8,440,225 residents (62.01%) from the 6 urban districts (Dongcheng, Xicheng, Chaoyang, Haidian, Fengtai, and Shijingshan; Chongwen and Xuanwu were merged into Dongcheng and Xicheng, respectively, in 2010) and 5,170,063 residents (37.99%) from the 10 peri-urban districts (Mentougou, Fangshan, Tongzhou, Shunyi, Changping,Daxing, Huairou, Pinggu, Miyun, and Yanqing).

1.3.2 Content of this annual report

The present annual report summarizes the data of the cancer incidence and mortality of all the permanent residents and the population data of the 16 districts in 2017 in Beijing. We report the quality control indicators in details, including the mortality to incidence ratio (M/I), the percentage of morphological verified cases (MV%), the percentage of cases recognized by the percentage of death certificate only (DCO%), and the percentage of "other and unspecified cases" (O&U%). We report data of new cases and deaths of all cancers and by 23 main sites, including crude incidence, mortality, age-standardized rates (ASRs) of the Chinese population in 2000, ASRs of Segi's world population, cumulative rates, age-specific rates, and sex-specific rates. Moreover, the characters of subsites and morphological sub-types for specific cancers were also calculated and described.

2 资料来源、方法与质量控制
Data source, collection methods and quality control

2.1 北京市以人群为基础的肿瘤登记资料收集方法

北京市肿瘤登记资料的收集采用被动和主动两种方法。被动收集是指各医院定期报送肿瘤病例资料，或肿瘤登记处从死因监测部门获取肿瘤患者死亡信息。主动收集是指到医院查阅肿瘤病例的诊疗病史，摘录肿瘤病历信息，或主动随访以获取癌症患者的生存信息。

2.1.1 北京市肿瘤登记资料的主要来源渠道

北京市 168 家二级及以上医疗机构（表 2.1.1）每月将住院肿瘤患者的发病和死亡信息通过"北京市卫生综合统计信息平台"报告至北京市肿瘤登记处。

死亡病例的主要来源为北京市疾病预防控制中心生命统计部门提供的肿瘤患者死亡数据库，同时作为补充肿瘤登记发病资料漏报的重要渠道。

对于数据库中仍存活病例（现患病例），将通过社区主动随访的形式进一步补充可能的死亡结局。

人口资料来源于北京市公安局的人口统计资料，标准人口结构来源于人口普查资料和 Segi 世界标准人口结构。

2.1 Methods of the data collection from population-base cancer registry of Beijing

We adopted passive and active data collection methods. Passive collection was defined as reporting of the information of the diagnosed cancer patients by the hospitals to the registry at regular intervals (for example, monthly in Beijing) or linking the data file of the vital statistics derived from the responsible department. Active collection happened when the registry retrieved the cancer data proactively from medical record departments of the hospitals, insurance bureaus and public security bureaus or followed up the cancer patients in the communities for the survival status.

2.1.1 Data sources of the Beijing cancer registry

Cancer incidence and mortality data from the 168 health institutions (secondary and above, Table 2.1.1) were submitted to the BCR monthly using the "Beijing Health-care Information Statistical Platform".

The death certificate data were derived from the cancer patient mortality database of the vital statistics department of Beijing Center for Diseases Prevention and Control. The database was used as an important supplementary source to improve the completeness of the data.

The patients that were still recorded as alive in the database were followed-up proactively at the community level.

The population data were provided by the Beijing Municipal Public Security Bureau. The standard age structure of the population was based on the China population census data and Segi's world standardized population structure.

表 2.1.1 2017 年北京市报告肿瘤登记资料医疗机构
Table 2.1.1 The medical institutions which submitted cancer case data in Beijing, 2017

辖区 Districts	医疗机构数 No. of medical institutions	医疗机构名单 List of medical institutions
北京市 Beijing	1	北京市疾病预防控制中心 Beijing Center for Diseases Prevention and Control
东城区 Dongcheng	16	中国医学科学院北京协和医院 Peking Union Medical College Hospital
		首都医科大学附属北京天坛医院 Beijing Tiantan Hospital, Capital Medical University
		北京医院 Beijing Hospital
		首都医科大学附属北京同仁医院 Beijing Tongren Hospital, Capital Medical University
		首都医科大学附属北京妇产医院 Beijing Obstetrics and Gynecology Hospital, Capital Medical University
		北京市普仁医院 Beijing Puren Hospital
		首都医科大学附属北京中医医院 Beijing Hospital of Traditional Chinese Medicine, Capital Medical University
		北京中医药大学东直门医院 Dongzhimen Hospital, Beijing University of Chinese Medicine
		首都医科大学附属北京口腔医院 Beijing Stomatological Hospital, Capital Medical University
		北京市第六医院 Peking University Sixth Hospital
		北京市隆福医院 Beijing Longfu Hospital
		北京同仁堂中医医院 Beijing Tongrentang Hospital of Traditional Chinese Medicine
		北京市和平里医院 Beijing Hepingli Hospital

续表

辖区 Districts	医疗机构数 No. of medical institutions	医疗机构名单 List of medical institutions
		北京市东城区第一人民医院 Beijing Dongcheng District First People's Hospital
		北京市东城区第一妇幼保健院 Beijing Dongcheng First Maternal and Child Health Hospital
		北京市鼓楼中医医院 Beijing Gulou Traditional Chinese Medicine Hospital
西城区 Xicheng	20	北京大学人民医院 Peking University People's Hospital
		北京大学第一医院 Peking University First Hospital
		首都医科大学附属北京友谊医院 Beijing Friendship Hospital, Capital Medical University
		首都医科大学宣武医院 Xuanwu Hospital, Capital Medical University
		首都医科大学附属北京儿童医院 Beijing Children's Hospital, Capital Medical University
		北京积水潭医院 Beijing Jishuitan Hospital
		中国中医科学院广安门医院 Guang'anmen Hospital, China Academy of Chinese Medical Sciences
		首都医科大学附属复兴医院 Fuxing Hospital, Capital Medical University
		北京市健宫医院 Beijing Jiangong Hospital
		北京市肛肠医院 Beijing Rectum Hospital
		北京市西城区展览路医院 Beijing Zhanlanlu Hospital
		北京市西城区广外医院 Guangwai Hospital of Xicheng District, Beijing
		北京市监狱管理局中心医院 Beijing Prison Administration Central Hospital
		北京市回民医院 Beijing Huimin Hospital

续表

辖区 Districts	医疗机构数 No. of medical institutions	医疗机构名单 List of medical institutions
		北京市第二医院 The Second Hospital of Beijing
		北京市宣武中医医院 Beijing Xuanwu Traditional Chinese Medical Hospital
		中国医学科学院阜外医院 Fuwai Hospital, Chinese Academy of Medical Sciences
		北京市丰盛中医骨伤专科医院 Beijing Fengsheng Special Hospital of Traditional Medical Traumatology and Orthopaedics
		北京新世纪儿童医院 New Century International Children's Hospital
		北京中医药大学附属护国寺中医医院 Huguosi Hospital of Traditional Chinese Medicine of Beijing University of Chinese Medicine
朝阳区 Chaoyang	31	中国医学科学院肿瘤医院 Cancer Hospital, Chinese Academy of Medical Sciences
		中日友好医院 China-Japan Friendship Hospital
		首都医科大学附属北京朝阳医院 Beijing Chao-Yang Hospital, Capital Medical University
		首都医科大学附属北京安贞医院 Beijing Anzhen Hospital, Capital Medical University
		首都医科大学附属北京地坛医院 Beijing Ditan Hospital, Capital Medical University
		煤炭总医院 Beijing Coal General Hospital
		北京华信医院 Beijing Huaxin Hospital
		中国医科大学航空总医院 Aviation General Hospital, China Medical University
		首都儿科研究所附属儿童医院 Children's Hospital, Capital Institute of Pediatrics
		民航总医院 Civil Aviation General Hospital

续表

辖区 Districts	医疗机构数 No. of medical institutions	医疗机构名单 List of medical institutions
		北京市垂杨柳医院 Beijing Chui Yang Liu Hospital
		中国中医科学院望京医院 Wangjing Hospital of China Academy of Chinese Medical Sciences
		北京中医药大学第三附属医院 Beijing University of Chinese Medicine Third Affiliated Hospital
		北京和睦家医院 Beijing United Family Hospital
		北京市第一中西医结合医院 Beijing First Integrated Traditional Chinese and Western Medicine Hospital
		北京市朝阳区妇幼保健院 Chaoyang District Maternal and Child Health Care Hospital
		北京五洲妇儿医院 GlobalCare Women and Children's Hospital
		北京市朝阳区双桥医院 Shuangqiao Hospital of Chaoyang District, Beijing
		北京朝阳急诊抢救中心 Beijing Chaoyang Emergency Medical Center
		北京市朝阳区桓兴肿瘤医院 Cancer Hospital of Huanxing ChaoYang District, Beijing
		中国藏学研究中心北京藏医院 Beijing Tibetan Hospital, China Tibetology Research Center
		北京精诚博爱康复医院 Beijing Jingcheng Boai Rehabilitation Hospital
		北京首都国际机场医院 Beijing Capital International Airport Hospital
		北京华府妇儿医院 Huafu Women and Children's Hospital
		北京百子湾和美妇儿医院 HarMoniCare Beijing Women and Children's Hospital
		北京玛丽妇婴医院 Beijing Mary's Hospital for Women and Children
		北京亚运村美中宜和妇儿医院 Amcare Women's and Children's Hospital
		北京优联耳鼻喉医院 Beijing Unicare EENT Hospital

辖区 Districts	医疗机构数 No. of medical institutions	医疗机构名单 List of medical institutions
		北京麦瑞骨科医院 Mary's Orthopedic Hospital, Beijing
		北京市红十字会急诊抢救中心 Red Cross Society of China Beijing Branch
		北京市老年病医院 Beijing Geriatrics Hospital
丰台区 Fengtai	23	首都医科大学附属北京佑安医院 Beijing Youan Hospital, Capital Medical University
		北京瑶医医院 Beijing Yao Medicine Hospital
		国家电网公司北京电力医院 Beijing Electric Power Hospital
		北京京西肿瘤医院 Western Beijing Cancer Hospital
		北京航天总医院 Beijing Aerospace General Hospital
		北京丰台医院 Beijing Fengtai Hospital
		北京中医药大学东方医院 Dongfang Hospital, Beijing University of Chinese Medicine
		中国航天科工集团七三一医院 Aerospace 731 Hospital
		北京博爱医院 Beijing Boai Hospital
		北京长峰医院 Beijing Changfeng Hospital
		北京市丰台中西医结合医院 Beijing Fengtai Hospital of Integrated Traditional and Western Medicine
		北京市丰台区南苑医院 Nanyuan Hospital, Fengtai District, Beijing
		北京市丰台区老年人协会莲花池康复医院 Beijing Lianhuachi Rehabilitation Hospital

续表

辖区 Districts	医疗机构数 No. of medical institutions	医疗机构名单 List of medical institutions
		北京市丰台区铁营医院 Tieying Hospital of Fengtai District Beijing
		北京丰台英博中西医结合医院 Beijing Fengtai Yingbo Hospital of Integrated Traditional and Western Medicine
		北京博仁医院 Beijing Boren Hospital
		北京丰台华山医院 Beijing Fengtai Huashan Hospital
		北京六一八厂医院 Beijing 618 Factory Hospital
		北京市丰台区妇幼保健计划生育服务中心 Beijing Fengtai Maternal and Child Health and Family Planning Service Center
		北京市木材厂职工医院 Beijing Timber Factory Worker's Hospital
		北京华坛中西医结合医院 Beijing Huatan Integrative Medicine Hospital
		北京市丰台区妇幼保健院 Fengtai Maternal and Child Health Hospital
		北京市红十字会和平医院 Beijing Red Cross Heping Hospital
石景山区 Shijingshan	7	北京大学首钢医院 Peking University Shougang Hospital
		北京市石景山医院 Beijing Shijingshan Hospital
		清华大学玉泉医院 Yuquan Hospital Affiliated to Tsinghua University
		首都医科大学附属北京康复医院 Beijing Rehabilitation Hospital of Capital Medical University
		中国中医科学院眼科医院 Eye Hospital, China Academy of Chinese Medical Sciences
		中国医学科学院整形外科医院 Plastic Surgery Hospital of Chinese Academy of Medical Sciences
		北京联科中医肾病医院 Beijing United-Tech Nephrology Specialist Hospital

续表

辖区 Districts	医疗机构数 No. of medical institutions	医疗机构名单 List of medical institutions
海淀区 Haidian	18	北京肿瘤医院 Beijing Cancer Hospital
		北京大学第三医院 Peking University Third Hospital
		首都医科大学附属北京世纪坛医院 Beijing Shijitan Hospital, Capital Medical University
		航天中心医院 Aerospace Center Hospital
		首都医科大学三博脑科医院 Sanbo Brain Hospital, Capital Medical University
		北京大学口腔医院 Peking University Hospital of Stomatology
		北京市海淀医院 Beijing Haidian Hospital
		中国中医科学院西苑医院 Xiyuan Hospital, China Academy of Chinese Medical Sciences
		北京市中关村医院 Beijing Zhongguancun Hospital
		北京老年医院 Beijing Geriatric Hospital
		北京市海淀区妇幼保健院 Haidian Maternal and Child Health Hospital
		北京水利医院 Beijing Water Conservancy Hospital
		北京市中西医结合医院 Beijing Hospital of Integrated Traditional Chinese and Western Medicine
		北京裕和中西医结合康复医院 Beijing Yuho Rehabilitation Hospital
		北京四季青医院 Beijing Sijiqing Hospital
		清华大学医院 Tsinghua University Hospital
		北京大学医院 Peking University Hospital
		北京德尔康尼骨科医院 Beijing Diakonie Orthopaedic Hospital

续表

辖区 Districts	医疗机构数 No. of medical institutions	医疗机构名单 List of medical institutions
门头沟区 Mentougou	4	北京京煤集团总医院 Beijing Jingmei Group General Hospital
		北京市门头沟区医院 Beijing Mentougou District Hospital
		北京市门头沟区妇幼保健院 Mentougou Maternal and Child Health Hospital
		北京市门头沟区中医医院 Beijing Mentougou Hospital of Traditional Chinese Medicine
房山区 Fangshan	7	北京市房山区第一医院 The Frist Hospital of Fangshan District, Beijing
		北京市房山区良乡医院 Liangxiang Hospital, Fangshan District, Beijing
		北京燕化医院 Beijing Yanhua Hospital
		北京市房山区中医医院 Fangshan District Hospital of Traditional Chinese Medicine of Beijing
		北京市房山区妇幼保健院 Fangshan District Maternal and Child Health Hospital
		中国核工业北京四〇一医院 Beijing 401 Hospital, China Nuclear Industry
		北京同济东方中西医结合医院 Beijing Tongji Oriental Hospital of Integrated Traditional and Western Medicine
通州区 Tongzhou	5	首都医科大学附属北京胸科医院 Beijing Chest Hospital, Capital Medical University
		首都医科大学附属北京潞河医院 Beijing Luhe Hospital, Capital Medical University
		北京市通州区中医医院 Tongzhou Traditional Chinese Medicine Hospital
		北京市通州区妇幼保健院 Tongzhou Maternal and Child Health Hospital of Beijing
		北京市通州区中西医结合医院 Tongzhou District Hospital of Integrative Medicine of Beijing
顺义区 Shunyi	5	北京市顺义区医院 The Hospital of Shunyi District, Beijing

续表

辖区 Districts	医疗机构数 No. of medical institutions	医疗机构名单 List of medical institutions
		北京市顺义区妇幼保健院 Shunyi District Maternal and Child Health Hospital, Beijing
		北京市顺义区中医医院 Beijing Shunyi Hospital of Traditional Chinese Medicine
		北京市顺义区空港医院 Beijing Shunyi Airport Hospital
		首都医科大学附属北京地坛医院顺义院区 Beijing Ditan Hospital, Capital Medical University (Shunyi)
昌平区 Changping	12	北京大学国际医院 Peking University International Hospital
		北京清华长庚医院 Beijing Tsinghua Changgung Hospital
		北京王府中西医结合医院 Beijing Royal Integrative Medicine Hospital
		北京市昌平区医院 Beijing Changping Hospital
		北京市昌平区中医医院 Chinese Medicine Hospital of Beijing Changping District
		北京京都儿童医院 Beijing Jingdu Children's Hospital
		北京市昌平区妇幼保健院 Changping Women and Children Health Care Hospital
		北京市昌平区中西医结合医院 Beijing Changping Hospital of Integrated Chinese and Western Medicine
		北京大卫中医医院 Beijing David Chinese Medicine Hospital
		北京市昌平区南口医院 Nankou Hospital of Changping District of Beijing
		北京小汤山医院 Beijing Xiaotangshan Hospital
		北京市昌平区沙河医院 Shahe Hospital, Changping District, Beijing
大兴区 Daxing	6	北京南郊肿瘤医院 Beijing Nanjiao Cancer Hospital
		北京市大兴区人民医院 Renmin Hospital of Daxing District, Beijing

续表

辖区 Districts	医疗机构数 No. of medical institutions	医疗机构名单 List of medical institutions
		北京市仁和医院 Beijing Renhe Hospital
		中国中医科学院广安门医院南区 Guang'anmen Hospital, China Academy of Chinese Medical Sciences (South)
		北京市大兴区中西医结合医院 Beijing Daxing District Hospital of Integrated Chinese and Western Medicine
		北京市大兴区妇幼保健院 Beijing Daxing Maternal and Child Care Hospital
怀柔区 Huairou	4	北京怀柔医院 Beijing Huairou Hospital
		北京市怀柔区中医医院 Huairou Hospital of Traditional Chinese Medicine
		北京市怀柔区妇幼保健院 Huairou District Maternal and Child Health Hospital
		北京康益德中西医结合肺科医院 Beijing Kangyide Integrated Traditional Chinese and Western Medicine Pulmonary Hospital
平谷区 Pinggu	4	北京市平谷区医院 Beijing Pinggu Hospital
		北京市平谷区中医医院 Beijing Pinggu Traditional Chinese Medicine Hospital
		北京市平谷岳协医院 Yuexie Hospital
		北京市平谷区妇幼保健院 Beijing Pinggu District Maternal and Children Health Care Institute
密云区 Miyun	3	北京市密云区医院 Hospital of Beijing Miyun District
		北京市密云区妇幼保健院 Maternal and Child Care Service Center of Miyun District in Beijing
		北京市密云区中医医院 Miyun District Hospital of Traditional Chinese Medicine
延庆区 Yanqing	3	北京市延庆区医院 Beijing Yanqing District Hospital
		北京中医医院延庆医院 Yanqing Hospital of Beijing Chinese Medicine Hospital
		北京市延庆区妇幼保健院 Yanqing Maternal and Child Health Care Hospital of Beijing

2.1.2 北京市肿瘤登记的数据管理及质控流程

肿瘤登记处收集肿瘤病例发病和死亡资料后，需要完成整理分类、查重、死亡补发病、病案核查、随访以及质量控制等环节，才能形成纳入年报分析的数据库。

首先，登记人员在"北京市卫生综合统计信息平台"定期整理医院报告的发病病例信息，根据患者的户籍地址区分本地和外地病例。本地患者纳入数据库，外地患者（约占60%）根据需要转给其他省级登记处。

然后，将当年发病的本地患者按照身份证、姓名和出生日期等关键变量与当年发病数据库查重，保存一条信息最全的发病信息，再与往年数据库中近百万例病例进行查重。未查询到重卡即按照新增病例统计；若发现重卡，先合并、补充和更新信息，然后再剔除重卡。

将历年的发病数据库与生命统计部门提供的死亡数据库匹配身份证号码，同一患者补充死亡时间和死因，如发病数据库查询不到对应的肿瘤死亡病例，提示可能存在漏报，及时追溯发病信息补报。

将当时仍显示存活的现患病例资料发给社区卫生服务中心开展主动随访工作。登记处应定期对存疑的病例开展病案核查工作。

最后，使用国际癌症研究署／国际肿瘤登记协会（International Agency for Research on Cancer/International Association of Cancer Registry,

2.1.2 Data management and quality control of the BCR

In order to meet the quality criteria of the data for the Annual Report publishing, we sorted and cleaned the data, identified duplicated cases, linked the cases in our registry with those in the survival status dataset by citizen ID number to obtain supplementary data and improve the completeness of data, re-abstracted the medical records, and followed up discharged patients after the registry collected the incidence and mortality data.

Firstly, the registrars, at regular intervals, sorted out the information of the new cases reported by the hospitals on the "Beijing Health-care Information Statistical Platform", and distinguished local and non-local cases according to the patient's permanent address. Information of local patients was included in the database. Data of the non-local patients (about 60% in the reported cases) were transferred to the registries in other provinces as needed.

In order to avoid duplication, the information of new cases diagnosed in the current year were linked to the database of the corresponding year, based on the key variables such as their citizen ID number, patient's name, and date of birth. Finally, the most complete entry of information of the patient would be saved, and then re-linked with the database (nearly one million cases) of previous years to find history duplicates. If not matched, the case would be included into the database as a new case of the current year. If the case was identified as duplicated, we would merge, supplement, and update the historic variable of this patient first, and then delete the information of the duplicated one.

The incidence database was linked with the mortality database provided by the vital statistics department by using the number of citizen ID card. We would supplement the date of death and the cause of the death for the same patient if the information from the two databases matched. If the data from the incidence database failed to match with the corresponding mortality data from the vital statistics department, it indicated that underreporting might have happened, and immediate make-up reporting would follow after tracing the incidence information.

IARC/IACR）的肿瘤登记工具软件（Cancer Registry Tools，IARCcrgTools 2.13） 中 的 Check 程序，对数据库逐一检查所有记录的变量是否完整和有效，同时对不同变量之间是否合乎逻辑的一致性进行检查。

2.1.3 北京市肿瘤登记重点工作

2.1.3.1 病案核查

形态学编码为 8000/3、8010/3 的病例，部位不明（other and unspecified, O&U）、仅有死亡医学证明书（death certificate only, DCO）和存在逻辑错误的病例，除外淋巴瘤、白血病等极易获取病理的癌种和肝、胆、胰等极难获得病理的癌种，其余病例均需根据病案号返回原报告医院查询病案首页、手术记录、病理报告、检查结果等病历信息，以核实诊断和户籍，补充病理诊断结果，查找肿瘤的具体解剖学部位。每年针对所有的儿童恶性肿瘤资料都开展病案核查，从而对病例进行再摘录和再编码工作。

2.1.3.2 病例随访

随访工作的开展采用被动随访和主动随访相结合的方式进行。肿瘤登记处首先将肿瘤发病库与全死因登记库进行被动匹配。未匹配上的患者与北京市卫生健康委员会信息统计中心的医院门诊数据库系统匹配身份证号码，1 年之内无门诊和住院记录的患者通过"北京市肿瘤患者随访信息系统"，由社区卫生服务中心 / 站采用电话或者入户的方式定期开展主动随访，获取病例的生存情况。

The data and information of the cases recorded as alive in the database would be sent to the community health service center for proactive follow-up. And the cancer registry would regularly carry out re-abstraction of medical records for suspected cases.

Finally, the software IARCcrgTools 2.13 provided by the International Agency for Research on Cancer/ International Association of Cancer Registry (IARC/ IACR) would be used to check whether all the collected variables were complete, accurate, and logically consistent.

2.1.3 Key Tasks of the BCR

2.1.3.1 Medical records re-verification

We would re-verify cases with the codes of 8000/3, 8010/3, O&U and DCO, and those with logical errors, except for cancers that are extremely easy to obtain the pathology, such as lymphoma and leukemia, and cancers that are extremely difficult to obtain the pathology, such as hepatobiliary cancer and pancreatic cancer. The cancer registrars would go to the reporting hospital, find the case by the medical record number at the medical record department of the hospital, and re-check the first-page information, surgical records, pathology reports and the findings of tests and investigations, and treatment outcomes in the medical records. A further re-verification would focus on whether the patients were local residents or not, their diagnostic and morphological information and the specific anatomical location of the tumor. All children malignant tumors were verified annually by re-extracting and re-coding the information of the medical records.

2.1.3.2 Patient follow-up

Both the passive and the active methods were used to follow the survival status of the patients. The registry's incidence database was linked with the death certificate database for patient identification using their citizen ID card number, then all unmatched cases were re-linked with the cases in the Beijing outpatient service database (within one year) provided by the statistical department of the Beijing Municipal Health Commission. Cases which were still unmatched would be followed-up at the community level by proactive methods, such as telephone calls or home visits.

2.2 北京市肿瘤登记资料收集内容

北京市肿瘤登记处收集北京市户籍人口、常住人口和来京就诊患者的全部恶性肿瘤、原位癌、中枢神经系统良性肿瘤及动态未定肿瘤病例（ICD-10 编码收集范围为 C00-97、D00-09、D32-33、D42-43、D45-47，年报统计范围为户籍人口 C00-97 和 D45-47）的发病、死亡和生存状态，以及北京户籍的相关人口资料。

2.2.1 新发病例资料

个人信息包括姓名、性别、出生日期、年龄、身份证号码、户籍地址、现住址、联系人、联系电话、民族、婚姻状况、职业等。肿瘤信息包括发病日期、解剖学部位（亚部位）、组织学类型、最高诊断依据、肿瘤分期等。转归结局包括是否死亡、死亡日期、死亡原因等。报告单位信息包括报告日期、病案号、报告单位、报告医生等（表 2.2.1）。

2.2 Items of patient information collected by the BCR

The BCR collected the data of new cases, mortality and survival status of the cases diagnosed with malignant tumors, carcinoma in situ, benign tumors of the central nervous system, and dynamic indeterminate tumors (ICD-10: C00-97, D00-09, D32-33, D42-43, D45-47. Cases with the codes of C00-97 and D45-47 were included into analysis in this annual report). The data cover the population of all the people with a Beijing household registration, permanent residents of Beijing, and residents of other provinces who visited Beijing for medical care.

2.2.1 Information of new cases

We collected the general information of the new cases, including the name, gender, date of birth, age, ID card number, permanent address, household address, contact person, contact person's telephone number, ethnicity, marital status, occupation; and the diagnostic information, including the incidence date, anatomical location (subsite), histological type, the most valid basis of diagnosis, tumor stage; and outcome information, including the survival status (death or not), date of death, cause of death; and the information of reporting hospital, including reporting date, medical record number, hospital name, the reporting doctor's name（Table 2.2.1）.

表 2.2.1 北京市肿瘤登记数据报告主要内容
Table 2.2.1 Main contents collected by Beijing Cancer Registry

序号 No.	数据采集项 Data collection item	数据类型 Data type	长度 Length	是否必填 If required	备注 Note
01	行政区划代码 Administrative division code	字符 String	6	是 Yes	
02	组织机构代码 Organization code	字符 String	9	是 Yes	各填报单位的组织机构代码 The organization code of each reporting unit
03	机构名称 Organization name	字符 String	200	是 Yes	

续表

序号 No.	数据采集项 Data collection item	数据类型 Data type	长度 Length	是否必填 If required	备注 Note
04	数据年份 Year of data	数字 Numeric	4	是 Yes	
05	数据月份 Month of data	数字 Numeric	2	是 Yes	1 至 12 1 to 12
06	填报人 Reporter name	字符 String	20	是 Yes	
07	填报日期 Reporting date	日期时间 Datetime	YYYY- MM-DD HH:MM:SS	是 Yes	
08	病案号 Medical record number	字符 String	20	是 Yes	
09	姓名 Name	字符 String	50	是 Yes	
10	性别代码 Sex	字符 String	1	是 Yes	
11	出生日期 Date of birth	日期 Date	YYYY- MM-DD	是 Yes	
12	年龄（岁） Age of diagnosis	数字 Numeric	3	否 No	
13	民族代码 Ethnic group	字符 String	2	否 No	
14	身份证号 Citizen ID card number	字符 String	18	否 No	15 或 18 位 15 or 18 bits
15	婚姻状况代码 Marital status	字符 String	1	是 Yes	
16	户籍省（直辖市、自治区） Household registration province (municipality, autonomous regions)	字符 String	50	否 No	
17	户籍市 Household registration city	字符 String	50	否 No	

序号 No.	数据采集项 Data collection item	数据类型 Data type	长度 Length	是否必填 If required	备注 Note
18	户籍县 Household registration county	字符 String	50	否 No	
19	户籍详细地址 Address of household registration	字符 String	200	肿瘤患者必填 Required for cancer patients	
20	户籍地址区编码 Household registration address district code	字符 String	6	肿瘤患者必填 Required for cancer patients	6 位代码 6 bits
21	户籍地址邮政编码 Household registration address postal code	字符 String	6	否 No	6 位数字 6 bits
22	现住址详细地址（居住半年以上） Current address (living for more than half a year)	字符 String	200	肿瘤患者必填 Required for cancer patients	
23	现住址省（直辖市、自治区）（居住半年以上） Current address province (municipality, autonomous regions)(living for more than half a year)	字符 String	50	否 No	
24	现住址市 Current address city	字符 String	50	否 No	
25	现住址区 Current address district	字符 String	50	否 No	
26	现住址区编码（居住半年以上） Current address district code (living for more than half a year)	字符 String	6	是 Yes	6 位代码 6 bits
27	现住址电话 Phone number	字符 String	20	否 No	
28	现住址邮政编码（居住半年以上） Current address postal code (living for more than half a year)	字符 String	6	否 No	6 位数字 6 bits
29	职业代码 Occupation code	字符 String	2	是 Yes	2 位职业代码 2 bits

续表

序号 No.	数据采集项 Data collection item	数据类型 Data type	长度 Length	是否必填 If required	备注 Note
30	工作单位及地址 Work unit's name and address	字符 String	200	否 No	
31	联系人姓名 Contact name	字符 String	50	否 No	
32	联系人地址 Contact address	字符 String	200	否 No	
33	联系人电话 Contact phone number	字符 String	20	否 No	
34	入院时间（时） Admission date	日期时间 Datetime	YYYY-MM-DD HH:MM:SS	是 Yes	
35	出院时间（时） Discharge date	日期时间 Datetime	YYYY-MM-DD HH:MM:SS	是 Yes	
36	出院时主要诊断编码 (ICD-10) Main diagnostic code at discharge (ICD-10)	字符 String	30	是 Yes	
37	出院主要诊断名称 Main diagnosis of discharge	字符 String	200	是 Yes	
38	入院病情 Admission condition	字符 String	1	是 Yes	
39	出院时其他诊断编码 (ICD-10) Other diagnostic code at discharge (ICD-10)	字符 String	30	是 Yes	
40	出院其他诊断名称 Other diagnosis of discharge	字符 String	200	是 Yes	
41	病理诊断编码（M 码） Pathological diagnostic code (M code)	字符 String	50	肿瘤患者必填 Required for cancer patients	
42	病理诊断名称 Pathological diagnosis name	字符 String	100	肿瘤患者必填 Required for cancer patients	
43	最高诊断依据代码 Code of the most valid basis of diagnosis	字符 String	1	肿瘤患者必填 Required for cancer patients	
44	分化程度编码 Differentiation code	字符 String	1	肿瘤患者必填 Required for cancer patients	

序号 No.	数据采集项 Data collection item	数据类型 Data type	长度 Length	是否必填 If required	备注 Note
45	肿瘤分期是否不详 Whether the tumor stage is unknown	字符 String	1	肿瘤患者必填 Required for cancer patients	
46	肿瘤分期 T Stage T	字符 String	1	"肿瘤分期是否不详"填"否"时，此项必填 When filling "No" in "whether the tumor stage is unknown", "Stage T" is required	
47	肿瘤分期 N Stage N	字符 String	1	"肿瘤分期是否不详"填"否"时，此项必填 When filling "No" in "whether the tumor stage is unknown", "Stage N" is required	
48	肿瘤分期 M Stage M	字符 String	1	"肿瘤分期是否不详"填"否"时，此项必填 When filling "No" in "whether the tumor stage is unknown", "Stage M" is required	
49	0 ～ IV 肿瘤分期 Stage 0 ～ IV	字符 String	1	"肿瘤分期是否不详"填"否"时，此项必填 When filling "No" in "whether the tumor stage is unknown", "Stage 0 ～ IV" is required	
50	主治医师姓名 Name of attending physician	字符 String	20	是 Yes	
51	离院方式代码 Discharge method code	字符 String	1	是 Yes	
52	死亡日期 Date of death	日期 Date	YYYY-MM-DD	否 No	
53	备注 Note	字符 String	500	否 No	

2.2.2 死亡资料

肿瘤死亡资料来源于全人群死因登记报告系统，包括根本死因、间接死因和其他死因涉及肿瘤原因的死亡资料。除身份证号码、户籍和出生日期等重要的个人信息外，还应包括死亡日期、死亡年龄、死亡原因主要诊断、诊断级别和依据、死亡地点等，根据填报的死亡医院和病案以及填报医生可以进一步追溯发病信息，降低仅有死亡医学证明书的比例（DCO%）。

2.2.3 随访资料

肿瘤病例随访资料包括最后接触时间、生存状态、死亡日期、死亡原因、是否失访、失访原因等。除此之外，北京市还对本人病情知晓情况、参加社区健康干预的意愿等进行登记。

2.2.4 人口资料

人口资料来源于北京市公安局逐年公布的人口资料。计算标化率所用的标准人口结构来源于2000年全国人口普查资料和 Segi 世界标准人口结构。人口资料包括居民人口总数及其性别、年龄别人口数或构成。年龄组按小于 1 岁（0~）、1~4 岁、5~9 岁、10~14 岁 …… 75~79 岁、80~84 岁、85 岁及以上（85+）分组。为计算肿瘤相对生存率，还需收集相应年份的寿命表。

2.3 北京市肿瘤登记质量控制指标

北京市肿瘤登记处根据《中国肿瘤登记工作指导手册（2016）》，参照 IARC/IACR《五大洲癌症发病率》第 XI 卷对肿瘤登记质量的有关要求，

2.2.2 Mortality data

The cancer mortality data, which included direct cause of death, indirect cause of death and other causes of death related to cancer, were derived from the population-based all causes of death surveillance database. We collected the general information such as patient's citizen ID number, permanent address, and date of birth, which helped to identify the patient, as well as the date of death, age at death, the main cause of death, the diagnostic basis of death and the place of death. The registrar would track the cases recognized by the death certificates for incidence variables according to the reporting hospital, the number of medical record, and the name of the reporting doctor to reduce the percentage of DCO (DCO%).

2.2.3 Follow-up data

The data collected through follow-up included date of last contact, survival status, date of death, causes of death, lost to follow-up or not, the reasons of lost to follow-up. In addition, the BCR also registered the patients' awareness of their disease and willingness to participate in community health interventions.

2.2.4 Population data

The population data were derived from the statistics released annually by the Beijing Municipal Public Security Bureau. The standard population structure used to calculate the standardized rate was derived from the 2000 national census data and Segi's world standardized population. The population data included the total number of permanent residents in Beijing and gender- and age- specific number of the population. They are divided into groups by age of 0-, 1-4, 5-9, 10-14··· 75-79, 80-84, 85+. In order to calculate the relative survival of cancer, life tables for the corresponding years were collected.

2.3 Criteria for data quality control

The data quality control criteria of the BCR was made according to the *Chinese Guideline for Cancer Registration,* and the *Cancer Incidence in Five Continents* volume XI by the International Agency for Research on Cancer (IARC) and International Association of Cancer Registries (IACR). The

从数据完整性、有效性和可比性等方面，制定了 MV%、M/I、DCO%、O&U% 等质量控制指标的标准，并且参考北京市历年的报告水平，要求北京市 MV%>75%、0.50<M/I<0.65、DCO%<2%、O&U%<10%，并参照此标准开展查漏补缺、病案核查和主动随访工作。

北京市肿瘤登记处在各个环节制定工作规范和质量控制程序，并严格执行，质量控制贯穿肿瘤登记工作的全过程。质量控制主要包括四个方面：完整性、有效性、可比性和时效性。

2.3.1 完整性

完整性是指在登记地区目标人群中发现所有发病病例的程度。常用的评价指标有死亡发病比（M/I）、DCO%、形态学确诊比例（MV%）、病例总数和不同来源的比例、每年发病率的稳定性、不同人群发病率的比较、年龄别发病率曲线、儿童肿瘤评价等。

2.3.1.1 死亡发病比（M/I）

死亡发病比是本年度的死亡病例数与发病病例数的比值。M/I 是用于评估肿瘤登记完整性的重要指标。M/I 过低说明存在死亡病例漏报、发病未查重或者随访工作质量差，M/I 过高说明发病存在漏报或者死亡补发病不完整，都与数据的完整性相关。

仅靠所有癌症合计的 M/I 值评估一个地区肿瘤登记的完整性并不准确。例如，我国大部分地区 M/I 介于 0.6~0.8 之间，但是北京市生存率高的甲状腺癌和乳腺癌患者所占比例大，就会拉低死亡病

completeness, comparability and validity of the data were evaluated using indicators such as MV%, M/I, DCO%, and O&U%. After taking the historical quality control data at BCR into consideration, the corresponding cutoff values and criteria for the indicators were set (MV%> 75%, 0.50<M/I<0.65, DCO%<2% and O&U%<10%) . The BCR carried out the quality control, re-abstraction of medical records and proactive follow-up based on the above criteria.

The BCR strictly implemented the guidelines and quality control procedures it had established in all processes. The quality control focused on four aspects: completeness, validity, comparability, and timeliness.

2.3.1 Completeness

The completeness of cancer registry data concerns about to what extent the new cases occurred in a defined population were registered in the cancer registration database. The indicators to evaluate the completeness included the mortality to incidence ratio (M/I), DCO%, MV%, the total number of registrations, the proportions of cases by reported sources, year-on-year incidence rate growth, and if possible, population-specific data, and age-specific data, for example, the incidence of childhood cancers and its year-on-year change.

2.3.1.1 Mortality to incidence ratio (M/I)

The M/I refers to the ratio of the number of deaths to the number of new cases in the current year. It is an important indicator for the assessment of the completeness of cancer registration data. If the M/I is too low, it indicates that the deaths may have been under-reported, that duplicated newly diagnosed cases exist, or the poor quality of follow-up; if the M/I is too high, it indicates that some new cases may have been under-reported or that there is incomplete recognition and supplementation of cases by death certificate.

It is not a good choice to evaluate the completeness of cancer data in a defined region based on the M/I value of all cancers. For example, the M/I of most areas in China was between 0.6 and 0.8. However, the M/I ratio of all cancers in Beijing was less than 0.55 due to the higher proportion of the patients with thyroid and breast cancers, both having a higher survival rate. Therefore,

例数，使 M/I 的比值不足 0.55，因此评估单癌种的 M/I 更为合理。

2.3.1.2 仅有死亡医学证明书的比例（DCO%）

DCO% 是指仅有死亡医学证明书的病例占所有癌症发病的比例，意味着患者生前没有肿瘤的诊疗记录或者无法获得诊疗信息，更不可能有形态学确诊的结果，病例的发病日期即死亡日期。死亡医学证明书是发现恶性肿瘤病例的有效补充途径，也是间接评价由死亡医学证明书发现病例比例（DCN%）的指标。DCO 病例是 DCN 追溯流程完成后的剩余部分，理论上应维持在一个恒定的较低比例，但不能为零。DCO% 是评价一个地区肿瘤登记资料完整性的重要指标。该指标过低，提示死亡补发病工作流程有误，未经治疗或者异地治疗的恶性肿瘤死亡病例未被补充到发病数据库中，存在漏报；DCO% 过高，则提示死亡病例未有效追溯发病信息，变量缺乏完整性。

2.3.1.3 形态学确诊比例（MV%）

形态学确诊（morphological verification, MV）的比例包括病理诊断和细胞学 / 血片诊断的病例所占百分比，既是完整性的指标，又是有效性的一个重要指标。IACR 建议 MV%>75%，但是该指标并不是越高越好，过高的形态学诊断比例说明病例均来源于医院报告，其他报告渠道可能存在漏报；过低的 MV% 也可能是未及时获取病理报告造成的，也可能是因为某一不易获取病理的癌种（例如肝癌）在所有癌种所占的比例较高所致，影响了数据的完整性。

it is more reasonable to evaluate the M/I of an individual cancer in a defined population.

2.3.1.2 Proportion of cases recognized by death certificate only (DCO%)

DCO% refers to the proportion of cases with death certificate only in all cancer cases, which means that the diagnosis and treatment information, such as the morphological type, was not available and the incidence date of the case is the same as the date of death. The death certification is an effective supplementation to find cancer cases, and it is also an indicator that could be used for indirect evaluation of the proportion of cases first notified by death certificate (DCN%). DCO cases are the remainder of cases after the identification of the new cases retrospectively by death certificates (DCN). Theoretically, the DCO should be maintained in a constantly lower level, but not zero. DCO% is an important indicator for evaluating the completeness of cancer registration data in a defined region. If DCO% is too low, it indicates that there might be problems in the process of identification of cases by death certificate: The case that received diagnosis and treatment in outpatient departments or received treatment out of the registration region were underreported or omitted. A too high DCO% means that the incidence information of death cases was not effectively traced, and the incidence data incomplete.

2.3.1.3 Proportion of morphologically verified cases (MV %)

The MV% refers to the percentage of cases diagnosed by pathology or cytology/hematology. It is an important indicator of both completeness and effectiveness of cancer registration data. The cutoff value of the MV% that IACR recommended was >75%. However, it's not the higher the better for this value. If the MV% is too high, it may indicate that the cases are all reported by hospitals, and there may be underreporting with the other reporting sources; if the MV% is too low, it may indicate that the results of the pathology were not reported in time. Another explanation for the excessively low MV% is that a relatively high proportion of a certain type of cancer (such as liver cancer) which is difficult to obtain pathology accounts for an excessively high proportion in all the cases, which also affects the completeness of the data.

$$MV\% = \frac{最高诊断依据为5、6、7、8的例数[1]}{报告肿瘤病例总例数} \times 100\%$$

$$MV\% = \frac{\text{The number of the patients with the most valid basis of diagnosis 5, 6, 7, 8}[2]}{\text{The total number of the patients}} \times 100\%$$

2.3.1.4 身份证号码的填写比例

鉴于肿瘤登记工作中复诊和随访的信息追溯都需要身份证号码作为关键变量，因此北京市非常重视身份证信息的收集和质控，医院上传的病例都需要校验身份证才能通过。2017年北京市肿瘤病例身份证的填写率达到98.87%。

2.3.2 有效性

有效性是指登记病例中具有给定特征（例如肿瘤部位、年龄、性别、诊断和编码）真正属性的病例所占的比例。再摘录与再编码方法是评价有效性最客观的方法，即通过再摘录与再编码核对符合程度以评估既往采集信息的准确率。

常用的评价指标有形态学确诊比例（MV%），仅有死亡医学证明书比例（DCO%）、部位不明比例（O&U%）。为保障有效性，北京市肿瘤登记处定期对身份证号码、出生日期、性别、继发或不明部位、无组织学诊断的病例开展病案记录核对、再摘录和再编码。

2.3.2.1 部位不明比例（O&U%）

肿瘤登记资料的有效性受错误和缺失资料的影

2.3.1.4 Proportion of cases that had filled in citizen ID card numbers

In view of the fact that the citizen ID card number is required as a key variable for re-abstraction of medical records and the follow-up, the BCR made great efforts to ensure the quality control of ID card number, which would help to improve the completeness of data. The citizen ID card number of all cancer cases uploaded to the on-line reporting system by hospitals needed to be verified. The proportion of cases that had filled in the numbers among the diagnosed cancer cases in Beijing reached 98.87% in 2017.

2.3.2 Validity

The validity refers to the proportion of registered cases with real attributes of a given characteristic (such as tumor location, age, gender, diagnosis, and code). In other words, to assess the accuracy of previously collected information and check the degree of conformity, re-extracting and re-coding would be conducted.

Commonly used evaluation indicators are MV%, DCO%, and O&U%. To ensure the accuracy, the BCR regularly re-extracts and re-codes the information of the patients, such as citizen ID card number, date of birth, gender, metastatic or unknown tumor sites, and cases without histological diagnosis.

2.3.2.1 Proportion of cases of other or unknown sites (O&U%)

The validity of cancer registration data is affected by reporting errors and missing items. At the same time,

---

1. 注：5，细胞学和血片；6，病理（继发）；7，病理（原发）；8，尸检（有病理）。

2. Notes：5，cytology or hematology；6，histology of metastasis；7，histology of primary；8，autopsy with concurrent or previous histology.

响。同时，由于受临床诊疗水平及患者依从性的客观影响，每年北京市肿瘤登记处都会收到报告继发和原发部位不详的病例，但历年的 O&U% 应该维持在相对较低的水平。

due to the doctor's clinical diagnosis and treatment capacity and patient compliance, the BCR would receive the reports of the cases with metastasis or cases with unknown primary sites each year. Ideally, the O&U% should be maintained at a relatively low level in a defined region.

$$O\&U\% = \frac{C26+C39+C48+C76\text{-}80+C97 \text{ 的例数}}{\text{报告肿瘤病例总例数}} \times 100\% \, [3]$$

$$O\&U\% = \frac{\text{The number of cases with the codes of } C26+C39+C48+C76\text{-}80+C97}{\text{The total number of patients}} \times 100\% \, [4]$$

2.3.2.2 形态学确诊比例（MV%）

MV% 是衡量数据有效性的一个重要指标。过低的 MV% 意味着大量的病例未经形态学诊断的确认，仅靠临床和影像等方式诊断，不排除有误诊病例混入的可能性。而且未经病理分型的病例资料，对其病因和预后因素的分析非常局限，会影响干预措施和卫生政策的制定，失去了肿瘤登记的目的和意义。

但是不同恶性肿瘤获取病理结果的难易程度不同，MV% 需要分癌种进行评估。例如肝癌和胰腺癌，由于病程短，发现时多数患者失去手术机会，其所在的解剖学位置也不易进行穿刺，因此 MV% 通常只有 20%~30%；相反，消化道的恶性肿瘤能通过内镜抓取活检组织获得病理结果，MV% 高达 99% 以上。因此，评估数据库的准确性不要局限于总体癌症的 MV%。

2.3.2.2 Proportion of morphologically verified cases (MV%)

The MV% is an important indicator to measure the validity of the data. If the MV% is too low, it means that a large number of cases were not been confirmed by microscopic diagnosis, and were confirmed by clinical and imaging evidence only, which risk the possibility of inaccurate diagnosis. Moreover, if a database included many cancer cases that were confirmed by non-microscopic evidence, it would hamper the researchers to explore the etiology and prognostic factors of cancer cases and mislead the health policy makers when they were to establish the intervention measures and health policies. In that case, cancer registration would become meaningless.

Nevertheless, the availability of pathological results for different tumors is quite different, so the MV% needs to be assessed by specific cancer types. For example, for liver and pancreatic cancers, due to the short course of disease, most patients would lose the opportunity for surgery when they were diagnosed, complicated by the difficulty for centesis due to the anatomical location of the organs, the MV% would stand at 20%-30%; on the contrary, tissues from the digestive tract can be biopsied easily by endoscopy,

---

3. 注：C26、C39、C48、C76-80 和 C97 均为 ICD-10 编码。C26，其他和不明确的消化系统恶性肿瘤；C39，呼吸和胸腔内器官其他和部位不明确的恶性肿瘤；C48，腹膜后和腹膜恶性肿瘤；C76-80，不明确、继发和未特指部位的恶性肿瘤；C97，独立的多个部位原发恶性肿瘤。

4. Note: ICD-10: C26, malignant neoplasm of other and ill-defined digestive organs; C39, malignant neoplasm of other and ill-defined sites in the respiratory system and intrathoracic organs; C48, retroperitoneal and peritoneal malignancies; C76-80, other, secondary malignant neoplasm of lymph nodes, respiratory and digestive organs and ill-defined sites; C97, malignant neoplasm of independent (primary) multiple sites.

2.3.2.3 仅有死亡医学证明书的比例（DCO%）

DCO% 是有效性的一个负面指标。DCO 意味着未作形态学诊断，因此 DCO% 过高会引起较低的 MV%，资料的有效性越差。但是前面也提到，由于客观条件的限制，DCO 无法避免，因此需要辩证地看待。此外，DCO% 过低也是不可信的。

2.3.3 可比性

数据结果可比的基本先决条件是采用通用的标准或定义。通常而言，可比性是指发病率间的不同不是因为各登记处之间的统计标准或数据质量不同而产生的。可比性涉及以下几个指标：对"发病"的定义，对原发、复发和转移的诊断标准，分类与编码，死亡证明等。

2.3.3.1 外部一致性

北京市肿瘤登记处收集资料的肿瘤部位编码采用ICD-10（International Statistical Classification of Diseases and Related Health Problems 10th Revision，ICD-10）编码，形态学编码采用ICD-O-2（International Classification of Diseases for Oncology, Second Revision, ICD-O-2）编码，整理过程中增加一列ICD-O-3（International Classification of Diseases for Oncology, Third Revision, ICD-O-3）编码。发病日期统一选择首次住院日期，多原发恶性肿瘤的判定采用IARC标准。中国标准人口年龄结构采用2000年全国人口普查资料，世界标准人口年龄结构采用Segi世界人口构成。

因此，比较各地区的恶性肿瘤发病、死亡和生存水平不应仅限报表数据的简单对比，还要结

therefore, the MV% of digestive tract tumors would stand as high as 99%. So, the accuracy of the data should not be evaluated by the MV% value of all the cancer sites, instead, the value of specific cancer sites should be used for the evaluation.

2.3.2.3 Proportion of death certificate only (DCO%)

The DCO% is a negative indicator of validity. DCO means that no information of morphological diagnosis has been collected. Therefore, a remarkably high DCO% will cause a lower MV%, and poor validity of the data. However, it has been mentioned earlier in the report that DCO cannot be avoided and should be viewed dialectically. If the DCO% is too low, it is unreliable too.

2.3.3 Comparability

The basic prerequisite for comparability of cancer registry data is the use of uniform standards or definitions. Generally speaking, comparability means that the difference in incidence rates in different regions or countries is not due to differences in statistical standards or data quality among the population-based registries. Comparability involves the following indicators: definition of "incidence"; diagnostic criteria for primary, recurrent and metastatic diseases; classification and coding; and death certificate, etc.

2.3.3.1 External Consistency

The coding of cancer site in the BCR uses the ICD-10, and the morphological coding ICD-O-2. A new code, the ICD-O-3 coding, which was transformed from ICD-O-2, was added in the process of data cleaning. The incidence date was defined as the date of first hospitalization, and the criteria of recognizing multiple primary malignancies was adopted using IARC standards. For Chinese standard age structure, we used the 2000 National Census data; and for the world's standard age structure, Segi's structure of the world population was used.

Therefore, comparison of the incidence, death, and survival levels of cancer cases in various regions should not be limited to simple comparison of the data reported in the Annual Reports, but should take the influencing factors into consideration. These factors include the

合该地区编码种类、收集范围、发病时间定义、多原发恶性肿瘤判断标准、标准人口结构等影响因素综合判断。

2.3.3.2 内部一致性

随访患者无准确死亡日期的，精确到年的记录为 7 月 1 日，精确到月的按 15 日登记。逻辑校验采用北京市报告系统自带的逻辑校验和有效性校验功能，包括年龄 / 出生日期、身份证有效性、性别 / 部位、性别 / 形态学、部位 / 形态学、最高诊断依据和形态学诊断的逻辑错误，日期一致性（死亡日期和随访日期不得早于发病日期，死亡日期不得早于随访日期等），编码一致性（发病编码和死亡编码的匹配）等，最后采用 IARCcrgTools 2.13 软件中的 Check 程序，对数据库病例逐一做最终检查。

2.3.4 时效性

时效性指肿瘤登记处收集、处理和发布完整及准确的肿瘤登记资料的及时性，一般指发病日期（诊断日期）到数据被利用时（年报、研究报告、政府发布、论文）的时间间隔。北京市各医院在患者出院 1 个月内报告病例资料，登记处需要等待 1 年完善患者的治疗及病理诊断结果。北京市疾病预防控制中心每年初提供上一年度的死亡病例数据库，登记处匹配死亡信息作为发病数据漏报的补充。由于大部分癌症患者的生存时间介于 1~3 年，因此死亡补发病工作持续 3 年才能补充完整；3 年期间每年定期随访患者，至少完成 1 次病案核查工作。

可见为保证数据的完整性和有效性，需要留给登记处足够的时间核实和补充资料，根据 IARC/

coding method, cases inclusion and exclusion criteria, definition of the incidence date, multiple primary tumor criteria, and standard age structure in the region.

2.3.3.2 Internal consistency

If a patient was followed up, but only the accurate death year was available, the deceased date of this patient would be recorded as July 1st, and if both the death year and month were available, the deceased date of the patient would be recorded as the 15th of the month. The logic verification process used the logic and validity check function of the BCR's reporting system. The verified contents included age/birth date, citizen ID validity, gender/tumor location, gender/morphology, tumor site/morphology, most valid basis of diagnosis and morphology diagnosis, date consistency (death date and follow-up date should not be earlier than incidence date, death date should not be earlier than last follow-up date, etc.), coding consistency (incidence code and death code matched or not), etc.; and a final check of all cases was performed using the software of IARCcrgTools 2.13.

2.3.4 Timeliness

Timeliness refers to the rapidity at which a registry can collect, finish quality control and publish reliable and complete cancer data. Generally, it refers to the time interval from the incidence date (date of first diagnosis) to the time when the data is used (for annual reports, government releases, research papers). Hospitals in Beijing would submit the information of new cancer cases within one month after the patient was discharged. The registry would need one year to do the quality control of the patient's treatment and pathological diagnosis results; the Beijing Center for Diseases Prevention and Control would provide the data of all cases of death of the previous year at the beginning of each year, and the BCR would link to this mortality database, using it as a supplementary source to detect the underreported cases. Since the survival time of most cancer patients was between 1-3 years, the supplementation could only be completed after 3 years, which would help the BCR to meet the criteria of completeness of cancer registration data; patients were followed up regularly every year during the above mentioned 3 years, and at least one medical record verification should be completed during the quality control period.

IACR 的建议，国际各登记处通常于诊断年份后的 3 年发布数据。

2.4 本肿瘤登记年报质量控制评价

2017 年，北京市肿瘤登记数据库的形态学确诊比例（MV%）为 78.13%，仅有死亡医学证明书比例（DCO%）为 0.08%，死亡发病比（M/I）为 0.52，部位不明比例（O&U%）为 1.93%（表 2.4.1）。

（撰稿　王宁，校稿　杨雷）

In order to ensure the completeness and validity of the data, it is necessary to leave enough time for cancer registries to verify and supplement the information. According to the recommendations of IARC/IACR, the registries around the world usually release data three years after the diagnosis year.

2.4 Data quality control of this annual report

The MV%, DCO%, M/I and O&U% of the cancer cases included for analysis in this annual report were 78.13%, 0.08%, 0.52 and 1.93%, respectively, in Beijing in 2017 (Table 2.4.1).

表 2.4.1 2017 年北京市肿瘤登记数据质量控制评价结果一览表
Table 2.4.1 Quality indicators of the cancer data in Beijing, 2017

部位 Site	全市 All			城区 Urban areas			郊区 Peri-urban areas		
	MV%	DCO%	M/I	MV%	DCO%	M/I	MV%	DCO%	M/I
口腔 Oral cavity & pharynx	82.88	0.00	0.52	84.10	0.00	0.47	80.00	0.00	0.63
鼻咽 Nasopharynx	65.00	0.00	1.08	68.75	0.00	1.31	59.38	0.00	0.72
食管 Esophagus	60.95	0.17	0.89	59.03	0.30	0.90	63.36	0.00	0.89
胃 Stomach	74.30	0.08	0.69	75.31	0.12	0.68	72.08	0.00	0.73
结直肠 Colon-rectum	85.69	0.05	0.48	85.17	0.07	0.49	86.85	0.00	0.45
肝 Liver	37.10	0.42	0.95	40.29	0.55	0.94	31.88	0.22	0.97
胆囊 Gallbladder	50.23	0.00	0.78	51.77	0.00	0.75	47.93	0.00	0.82
胰腺 Pancreas	31.30	0.00	0.93	30.32	0.00	0.95	33.41	0.00	0.90
喉 Larynx	84.19	0.00	0.43	85.14	0.00	0.40	82.76	0.00	0.48
肺 Lung	63.01	0.16	0.73	64.07	0.17	0.71	61.16	0.14	0.76

续表

部位 Site	全市 All			城区 Urban areas			郊区 Peri-urban areas		
	MV%	DCO%	M/I	MV%	DCO%	M/I	MV%	DCO%	M/I
骨 Bone	64.63	0.00	0.69	68.42	0.00	0.53	59.42	0.00	0.91
皮肤（黑色素瘤） Skin(melanoma)	100.00	0.00	0.73	100.00	0.00	0.68	100.00	0.00	0.87
乳腺 Breast	97.07	0.02	0.21	96.87	0.03	0.21	97.47	0.00	0.20
子宫颈 Cervix	85.43	0.31	0.36	87.47	0.51	0.36	82.38	0.00	0.37
子宫体 Uterus	94.85	0.00	0.18	94.26	0.00	0.20	95.84	0.00	0.14
卵巢 Ovary	84.56	0.00	0.56	86.58	0.00	0.58	80.87	0.00	0.52
前列腺 Prostate	85.93	0.00	0.38	86.77	0.00	0.38	83.53	0.00	0.38
睾丸 Testis	94.87	0.00	0.18	92.86	0.00	0.21	100.00	0.00	0.09
肾 Kidney	87.57	0.00	0.36	87.75	0.00	0.38	87.17	0.00	0.31
膀胱 Bladder	89.00	0.00	0.41	89.13	0.00	0.41	88.70	0.00	0.42
脑 Brain	71.17	0.15	0.75	77.00	0.25	0.74	62.41	0.00	0.76
甲状腺 Thyroid	98.78	0.00	0.02	98.73	0.00	0.02	98.87	0.00	0.02
淋巴瘤 Lymphoma	99.58	0.00	0.65	99.80	0.00	0.63	99.12	0.00	0.68
白血病 Leukemia	100.00	0.00	0.71	100.00	0.00	0.75	100.00	0.00	0.66
其他 Others	75.90	0.09	0.49	73.79	0.07	0.52	79.88	0.12	0.43
合计 **All sites**	78.13	0.08	0.52	78.93	0.10	0.51	76.58	0.05	0.53

3 统计分类指标释义
Interpretation of Statistical Items Classification

3.1 统计分类

3.1.1 癌症分类

参照国际上常用的癌症 ICD-10 分类统计表，根据 ICD-10 前三位"C"类编码，将癌症细分类为 59 部位、26 大类，真性红细胞增多症（D45）、骨髓增生异常综合征（D46）、淋巴造血和有关组织动态未定肿瘤（D47）归入髓样白血病。详见表 3.1.1 和表 3.1.2。

3.1 Items Classification

3.1.1 Cancer classification

Based on the ICD-10 classification principles, neoplasms were subdivided into 59 main sites, correspondent to 26 categories according to the first three number of the "C" codes. Polycythemia vera (D45), myelodysplastic syndrome (D46) and lymphoid, hematopoietic, and related tissue tumors with uncertain behavior (D47) were classified as myeloid leukemia in data analysis. See details on Table 3.1.1 and Table 3.1.2.

表 3.1.1 常用癌症分类统计表（细分类）
Table 3.1.1 Detailed cancer classification of ICD-10

部位 Site	ICD-10
唇 Lip	C00
舌 Tongue	C01-02
口 Mouth	C03-06
唾液腺 Salivary glands	C07-08
扁桃腺 Tonsil	C09
其他口咽 Other oropharynx	C10
鼻咽 Nasopharynx	C11
下咽 Hypopharynx	C12-13
咽，部位不明 Pharynx unspecified	C14
食管 Esophagus	C15
胃 Stomach	C16

部位 Site	ICD-10
小肠 Small intestine	C17
结肠 Colon	C18
直肠 Rectum	C19-20
肛门 Anus	C21
肝 Liver	C22
胆囊及其他 Gallbladder etc.	C23-24
胰腺 Pancreas	C25
鼻、鼻窦及其他 Nose, sinuses etc.	C30-31
喉 Larynx	C32
气管、支气管、肺 Trachea, bronchus & lung	C33-34
其他胸腔器官 Other thoracic organs	C37-38
骨 Bone	C40-41
皮肤（黑色素瘤）Skin (melanoma)	C43
皮肤（其他）Skin (other)	C44
间皮瘤 Mesothelioma	C45
卡波西肉瘤 Kaposi sarcoma	C46
周围神经、其他结缔组织和软组织 peripheral nerves, other connective & soft tissue	C47, C49
乳腺 Breast	C50
外阴 Vulva	C51
阴道 Vagina	C52
子宫颈 Cervix uteri	C53
子宫体 Corpus uteri	C54
子宫，部位不明 Uterus unspecified	C55
卵巢 Ovary	C56
其他女性生殖器 Other female genital organs	C57

部位 Site	ICD-10
胎盘 Placenta	C58
阴茎 Penis	C60
前列腺 Prostate	C61
睾丸 Testis	C62
其他男性生殖器 Other male genital organs	C63
肾 Kidney	C64
肾盂 Renal pelvis	C65
输尿管 Ureter	C66
膀胱 Bladder	C67
其他泌尿器官 Other urinary organs	C68
眼 Eye	C69
脑、神经系统 Brain, nervous system	C70-72
甲状腺 Thyroid	C73
肾上腺 Adrenal gland	C74
其他内分泌腺 Other endocrine	C75
霍奇金淋巴瘤 Hodgkin lymphoma	C81
非霍奇金淋巴瘤 Non-Hodgkin lymphoma	C82-85, C96
免疫增生性疾病 Immunoproliferative diseases	C88
多发性骨髓瘤 Multiple myeloma	C90
淋巴样白血病 Lymphoid leukemia	C91
髓样白血病 Myeloid leukemia	C92-94, D45-47
白血病，未特指 Leukemia unspecified	C95
其他或未指明部位 Other and unspecified（O&U）	C26,C39,C48,C76-80,C97
所有部位合计 All sites	**C00-97**
所有部位除外 C44 All sites except C44	**C00-97 exc. C44**

表 3.1.2 常用癌症分类统计表（大分类）
Table 3.1.2 Broad cancer classification of ICD-10

部位全称 Full name of site	部位简称 Short name of site	ICD-10
口腔和咽喉（除外鼻咽）Oral cavity & pharynx exc. nasopharynx	口腔 Oral cavity & pharynx	C00-10, C12-14
鼻咽 Nasopharynx	鼻咽 Nasopharynx	C11
食管 Esophagus	食管 Esophagus	C15
胃 Stomach	胃 Stomach	C16
结、直肠、肛门 Colon, rectum & anus	结直肠 Colon-rectum	C18-21
肝 Liver	肝 Liver	C22
胆囊及其他 Gallbladder and others	胆囊 Gallbladder	C23-24
胰腺 Pancreas	胰腺 Pancreas	C25
喉 Larynx	喉 Larynx	C32
气管、支气管、肺 Trachea, bronchus & lung	肺 Lung	C33-34
其他胸腔器官 Other thoracic organs	其他胸腔器官 Other thoracic organs	C37-38
骨 Bone	骨 Bone	C40-41
皮肤黑色素瘤 Melanoma of skin	皮肤黑色素瘤 Melanoma of skin	C43
乳房 Breast	乳房 Breast	C50
子宫颈 Cervix uteri	子宫颈 Cervix	C53
子宫体及子宫部位不明 Uterus & unspecified	子宫体 Uterus	C54-55
卵巢 Ovary	卵巢 Ovary	C56
前列腺 Prostate	前列腺 Prostate	C61
睾丸 Testis	睾丸 Testis	C62
肾及泌尿系统部位不明 Kidney & unspecified urinary organs	肾 Kidney	C64-66, C68
膀胱 Bladder	膀胱 Bladder	C67
脑、神经系统 Brain, nervous system	脑 Brain	C70-C72

部位全称 Full name of site	部位简称 Short name of site	ICD-10
甲状腺 Thyroid	甲状腺 Thyroid	C73
淋巴瘤 Lymphoma	淋巴瘤 Lymphoma	C81-85, C88, C90, C96
白血病 Leukemia	白血病 Leukemia	C91-95, D45-47
其他或未指明部位 Other and unspecified	其他或未指明部位（O&U）	C26,C39,C48,C76-80,C97
所有部位合计 All sites	合计 All sites	C00-97

3.1.2 城区和郊区分类

城区包括东城、西城、朝阳、海淀、丰台、石景山，郊区包括门头沟、房山、通州、顺义、昌平、大兴、怀柔、平谷、密云、延庆。

3.2 常用统计指标

3.2.1 年均人口数

年均人口数是计算发病（死亡）率指标的分母，精确算法是一年内每一天暴露于发病（死亡）危险的生存人数之和除以年内天数，但实际上很难掌握每一天的生存人数，因而常用年初和年末人口数的算术平均数作为年均人口数的近似值。

$$年均人口数（人）= \frac{年初（上年末）人口数 + 年末人口数}{2}$$

年中人口数指 7 月 1 日零时人口数，如果人口数变化均匀，年中人口数等于年均人口数，可以用年中人口数代替年均人口数。

3.1.2 Definition of urban and peri-urban areas

The urban areas of Beijing include Dongcheng, Xicheng, Chaoyang, Haidian, Fengtai, and Shijingshan; and the peri-urban areas include Mentougou, Fangshan, Tongzhou, Shunyi, Changping, Daxing, Huairou, Pinggu, Miyun, and Yanqing.

3.2 Statistical indicators

3.2.1 Average annual population

Average annual population is the denominator used in the calculation of the incidence (mortality) rates. Its theoretical value is the number of persons at risk of incidence (death) each day in a specific year divided by number of the days in the year. Considering the complexity of such calculation, we would often use the estimation/calculation as expressed by the following formula:

$$Average\ annual\ population = \frac{population\ at\ the\ end\ of\ the\ year\ + population\ in\ the\ beginning\ of\ the\ year}{2}$$

The number of mid-year population refers to the number of the population on 1st July at 00:00 AM. If the number of the population is relatively stable, the mid-year population could be used to represent average

3.2.2 性别、年龄别人口数

根据北京市公安局年末提供的户籍人口分性别百岁表计算。年龄的分组，规定除 0 岁组和 1~4 岁组以外，以间隔 5 岁为一组，即：0~、1~4、5~9、10~14…75~79、80~84、85+，共计 19 组。

3.2.3 发病（死亡）率

发病（死亡）率又称为粗发病（死亡）率，是反映人口发病（死亡）情况最基本的指标，是指某年该地登记的每 10 万人口癌症新病例（死亡）数，反映人口发病（死亡）水平。

$$发病（死亡）率（1/10 万）= \frac{某年某地癌症新病例（死亡）数}{某年某地年均人口数} \times 100\,000/10\,万$$

3.2.4 性别、年龄别发病（死亡）率

性别和年龄结构是影响恶性肿瘤发病（死亡）水平的重要因素。性别、年龄别发病（死亡）率是统计研究的重要指标。

$$某性别（年龄别）发病（死亡）率（1/10 万）= \frac{某性别（年龄组）发病（死亡）人数}{同性别（年龄组）人口数} \times 100\,000/10\,万$$

3.2.5 年龄调整率（标化率）

由于粗发病（死亡）率受人口年龄构成的影响较大，因此在对比分析不同地区的发病（死亡）率或同一地区人群不同时期的发病（死亡）水平时，为消除人口年龄结构对发病（死亡）水平的影响，

annual population.

3.2.2 Sex- and age-specific population

The sex-and age-specific population is provided by the Beijing Municipal Public Security Bureau. People were divided into 19 age groups of 0-, 1-4, 5-9, 10-14… 75-79, 80-84, 85+ years, respectively.

3.2.3 Incidence (mortality) rates

The incidence (mortality) rate is a measure of the frequency at which an event, such as a new case of cancer (cancer death), occurs in a population over a period of time.

$$Incidence\ (mortality)rate\ per\ 100,000 = \frac{new\ cases\ (new\ cancer\ death)\ occurred\ during\ a\ given\ time\ period}{population\ at\ risk\ at\ the\ same\ period} \times 100,000$$

3.2.4 Sex- and age-specific incidence (mortality) rates

Sex and age structure are important factors influencing the cancer incidence and mortality. Sex- and age-specific rates are important statistical indicators in cancer epidemiology.

$$Sex\text{-}\ or\ age\text{-}specific\ incidence\ (mortality)\ rate\ per\ 100,000 = \frac{cases\ in\ a\ specific\ sex\ or\ age\ group}{average\ number\ of\ population\ in\ the\ sex\ or\ age\ group} \times 100,000$$

3.2.5 Age standardized rates (ASRs)

Because the crude incidence (mortality) rate would be substantially affected by the age structure of the population, when comparing the incidence (mortality) rate in different regions or in the same region but at different periods of time, in order to eliminate the influence of the population's age structure on the incidence or mortality, it is necessary to calculate the age-standardized incidence (mortality) rate (ASIR or ASMR). In other words, the ASIR or ASMR

需要计算按年龄标准化发病（死亡）率，即指按照某一标准人口的年龄结构所计算的发病（死亡）率。本年报使用的中国标准人口是 2000 年全国第五次人口普查的人口构成（简称：中标率），世界标准人口采用 Segi 世界标准人口构成（简称：世标率）。表 3.2.1 为中国人口和世界人口年龄构成，可供计算年龄标化率时选用。

represents the incidence (mortality) rate after adjusting of age by a standardized age structure of a certain population. The Chinese standard population used in this annual report adopts the age structure of the fifth national census in 2000, and the world standard population adopts Segi's standard population structure. Table 3.2.1 shows the age structures of the Chinese and the world standard population, which could be used when calculating the age standardized rates.

表 3.2.1 标准人口构成
Table 3.2.1 Standard population

年龄组（岁） Age group(years)	中国人口构成（2000 年） Number of persons in Chinese standard population (2000)	世界人口构成 Number of persons in Segi's population
0~	13 793 799	2 400
1~4	55 184 575	9 600
5~9	90 152 587	10 000
10~14	125 396 633	9 000
15~19	103 031 165	9 000
20~24	94 573 174	8 000
25~29	117 602 265	8 000
30~34	127 314 298	6 000
35~39	109 147 295	6 000
40~44	81 242 945	6 000
45~49	85 521 045	6 000
50~54	63 304 200	5 000
55~59	46 370 375	4 000
60~64	41 703 848	4 000
65~69	34 780 460	3 000
70~74	25 574 149	2 000
75~79	15 928 330	1 000
80~84	7 989 158	500
85+	4 001 925	500
合计	1 242 612 226	100 000

年龄标化发病（死亡）率的计算（直接法）：

（1）计算年龄组发病（死亡）率。

（2）以各年龄组发病（死亡）率乘相应的标准人口年龄构成百分比，得到相应的理论发病（死亡）率。

（3）各年龄组的理论发病（死亡）率相加之和即为年龄标化发病（死亡）率。

$$\text{标化发病（死亡）率（1/10万）} = \frac{\Sigma\,[\text{标准人口各年龄组人口数或构成比}\times\text{年龄别发病（死亡）率}]}{\Sigma\,\text{标准人口各年龄组人口数或构成比}}$$

3.2.6 分类构成比

各类癌症发病（死亡）构成比可以反映各类恶性肿瘤对居民健康危害的情况。恶性肿瘤发病（死亡）分类构成比的计算公式如下：

$$\text{某恶性肿瘤构成比（\%）} = \frac{\text{某恶性肿瘤发病（死亡）人数}}{\text{恶性肿瘤总发病（死亡）人数}}\times100\%$$

3.2.7 累积发病（死亡）率

累积发病（死亡）率是指某病在某一年龄阶段内按年龄（岁）进行累积的发病（死亡）率总指标。累积发病（死亡）率消除了年龄构成不同的影响，故不需要标准化便可以直接用于不同地区的比较。恶性肿瘤一般是计算 0~74 岁的累积发病（死亡）率。

$$\text{累积发病（死亡）率（\%）} = (\Sigma\,[\text{年龄组发病（死亡）率}\times\text{年龄组距}])\times100\%$$

Direct method in calculating age-standardized incidence (mortality) rate:

(1) Calculate the rate for cases in a specific age group in a target population.

(2) Calculate the weighted age-specific rates. The weights applied represent the relative age distribution of the standard population.

(3) Add up each weighted age-specific rate. The sum of rates reflects the adjusted rate.

$$\text{ASR per 100,000} = \frac{\Sigma\,\text{standard population in corresponding age group}\times\text{age-specific rate}}{\Sigma\,\text{standard population}}$$

3.2.6 Relative frequency

The relative frequency indicates the percentage of the number of site-specific new cancer cases accounting in the numbers of all cancers combined. The formula is:

$$\text{Relative frequency of a certain type of cancer (\%)} = \frac{\text{No. of cases of a particular cancer}}{\text{No. of cases of all cancers}}\times100\%$$

3.2.7 Cumulative rate

A cumulative rate indicates the probability of the onset of a cancer between birth and a specific age. The cumulative incidence (death) rate eliminates the influence of age structure, so it can be directly compared in different regions without standardization. A cumulative rate is often calculated for population between 0 and 74 years.

$$\text{Cumulative rate(\%)} = [\,\Sigma\,(\text{age-specific rate}\times\text{width of the age groups})\,]\times100\%$$

（撰稿 王宁，校稿 杨雷）

4 2017 年北京市恶性肿瘤发病与死亡
Incidence and mortality for cancers in Beijing, 2017

4.1 北京市覆盖人口

2017 年北京市年中户籍人口数为 13 610 288 人（男性 6 791 497 人，女性 6 818 791 人）。其中，城区人口 8 440 225 人（男性 4 209 664 人，女性 4 230 561 人），占全市人口的 62.01%；郊区人口 5 170 063 人（男性 25 81 833 人，女性 2 588 230 人），占全市人口的 37.99%（表 4.1.1，图 4.1.1 至图 4.1.3 ）。

4.1 Population coverage in Beijing

In 2017, the number of mid-year population with household registration of Beijing was 13,610,288 (6,791,497 for males and 6,818,791 for females), for urban areas 8,440,225 (4,209,664 for males and 4,230,561 for females), or 62.01% of the total; and for peri-urban areas 5,170,063 (2,581,833 for males and 2,588,230 for females), or 37.99% of total (Table 4.1.1, Figure 4.1.1–4.1.3).

表 4.1.1 2017 年北京市肿瘤登记覆盖人口
Table 4.1.1 Population in different areas of Beijing in 2017

年龄组 Age group (years)	全市 All areas			城区 Urban areas			郊区 Peri-urban areas		
	男性 Male	女性 Female	合计 All	男性 Male	女性 Female	合计 All	男性 Male	女性 Female	合计 All
合计 Total	6 791 497	6 818 791	13 610 288	4 209 664	4 230 561	8 440 225	2 581 833	2 588 230	5 170 063
0~	82 433	77 226	159 659	45 073	42 143	87 216	37 360	35 083	72 443
1~	311 245	291 913	603 158	190 426	177 900	368 326	120 819	114 013	234 832
5~	293 664	274 774	568 438	183 768	171 562	355 330	109 896	103 212	213 108
10~	193 196	181 169	374 365	113 374	105 870	219 244	79 822	75 299	155 121
15~	217 457	213 525	430 982	131 913	131 157	263 070	85 544	82 368	167 912
20~	336 357	338 177	674 534	217 608	223 440	441 048	118 749	114 737	233 486
25~	504 147	489 340	993 487	295 211	285 131	580 342	208 936	204 209	413 145
30~	586 830	582 021	1 168 851	349 770	347 577	697 347	237 060	234 444	471 504
35~	537 302	529 873	1 067 175	340 386	339 650	680 036	196 916	190 223	387 139
40~	425 646	415 328	840 974	261 008	254 442	515 450	164 638	160 886	325 524
45~	543 363	539 143	1 082 506	314 685	314 902	629 587	228 678	224 241	452 919

年龄组 Age group (years)	全市 All areas			城区 Urban areas			郊区 Peri-urban areas		
	男性 Male	女性 Female	合计 All	男性 Male	女性 Female	合计 All	男性 Male	女性 Female	合计 All
55~	550 222	543 492	1 093 714	351 654	343 656	695 310	198 568	199 836	398 404
60~	544 499	572 571	1 117 070	347 007	363 281	710 288	197 492	209 290	406 782
65~	356 978	378 289	735 267	223 413	232 432	455 845	133 565	145 857	279 422
70~	219 629	247 797	467 426	133 756	151 812	285 568	85 873	95 985	181 858
75~	188 696	228 152	416 848	127 008	159 981	286 989	61 688	68 171	129 859
80~	166 994	187 206	354 200	122 972	138 103	261 075	44 022	49 103	93 125
85+	123 546	139 693	263 239	98 340	106 103	204 443	25 206	33 590	58 796

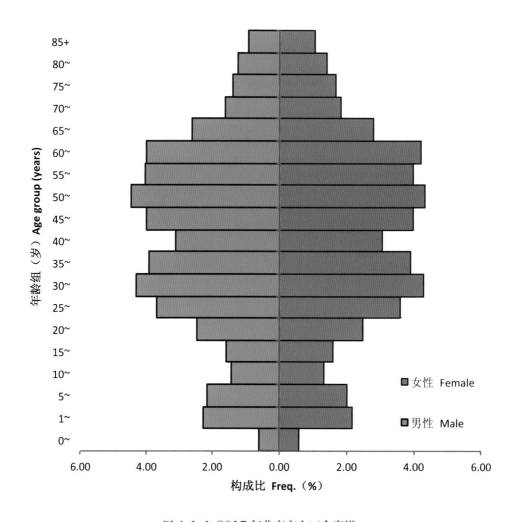

图 4.1.1 2017 年北京市人口金字塔

Figure 4.1.1 Population pyramid in Beijing, 2017

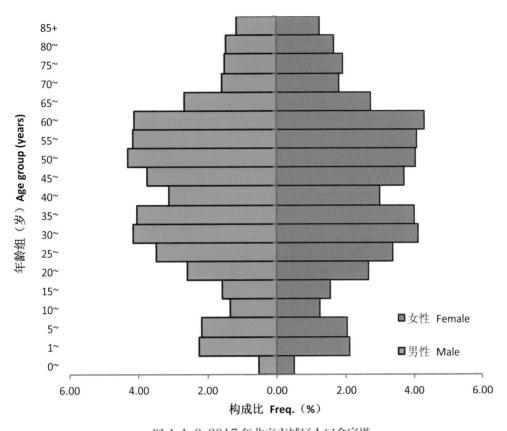

图 4.1.2 2017 年北京市城区人口金字塔
Figure 4.1.2 Population pyramid in urban areas of Beijing, 2017

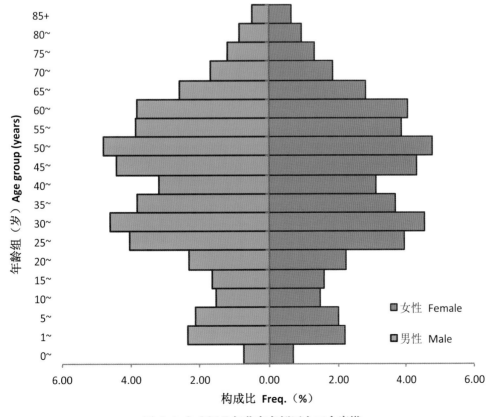

图 4.1.3 2017 年北京市郊区人口金字塔
Figure 4.1.3 Population pyramid in peri-urban areas of Beijing, 2017

4.2 北京市全部恶性肿瘤发病和死亡

4.2.1 北京市全部恶性肿瘤发病情况

2017 年北京市新发病例数 50 070 例（男性 24 752 例，女性 25 318 例），其中城区新发病例数为 32 997 例，占 65.90%，郊区 17 073 例，占 34.10%。全市发病率为 367.88/10 万（男性 364.46/10 万，女性 371.30/10 万），中标发病率为 200.42/10 万，世标发病率为 192.12/10 万，0~74 岁累积发病率为 21.27%。城区发病率为 390.95/10 万（男性 382.76/10 万，女性 399.10/10 万），中标发病率为 205.63/10 万，世标发病率为 196.71/10 万，0~74 岁累积发病率为 21.79%。郊区发病率为 330.23/10 万（男性 334.61/10 万，女性 325.86/10 万），中标发病率为 192.15/10 万，世标发病率为 184.87/10 万，0~74 岁累积发病率为 20.46%。城区与郊区相比，城区男性和女性发病率、中标发病率和世标发病率均高于郊区相应指标，城区男性 0~74 岁累积发病率低于郊区，但城区女性 0~74 岁累积发病率高于郊区（表 4.2.1）。

北京市全部恶性肿瘤世标发病率由 2008 年的 160.21/10 万上升到 2017 年的 192.12/10 万，年均变化百分比为 2.11%（*P*<0.001）；男性和女性发病 10 年间年均变化百分比分别为 0.96%（*P*=0.005）和 3.26%（*P*<0.001）。

4.2 Incidence and mortality for all cancer sites in Beijing

4.2.1 Incidence of all cancer sites in Beijing

In 2017, there were 50,070 new cases (24,752 for males and 25,318 for females) in Beijing, 32,997 (65.90%) in urban areas and 17,073 (34.10%) in peri-urban areas. The incidence rate of all cancers was 367.88 per 100,000 (364.46 per 100,000 for males and 371.30 per 100,000 for females), with an ASR China of 200.42 per 100,000, an ASR World of 192.12 per 100,000, and a cumulative rate for subjects aged 0 to 74 years of 21.27%. The incidence rate of all cancers in urban areas was 390.95 per 100,000 (382.76 per 100,000 for males and 399.10 per 100,000 for females), with an ASR China of 205.63 per 100,000, an ASR World of 196.71 per 100,000, and a cumulative rate for subjects aged 0 to 74 years of 21.79%. The incidence rate of all cancer sites in peri-urban areas was 330.23 per 100,000 in 2017 (334.61 per 100,000 for males and 325.86 per 100,000 for females), with an ASR China of 192.15 per 100,000, an ASR World of 184.87 per 100,000, and a cumulative incidence rate for subjects aged 0 to 74 years of 20.46%. The crude incidence rates, ASR China for incidence, and ASR world for incidence of all cancer sites were higher in urban areas than those in peri-urban areas for both sexes. The cumulative incidence rate was higher in peri-urban areas than that in urban areas for males, but lower in peri-urban areas than that in urban areas for females (Table 4.2.1).

The ASR World for incidence of all cancers in Beijing increased from 160.21 per 100,000 in 2008 to 192.12 per 100,000 in 2017; the annual percentage change (APC) was 2.11% (*P*<0.001). And the APCs in the last 10 years for males and females were 0.96% (*P*=0.005) and 3.26% (*P*<0.001), respectively.

表 4.2.1 2017 年北京市户籍居民全部恶性肿瘤发病情况
Table 4.2.1 Incidence of all cancer sites in Beijing, 2017

地区 Areas	性别 Sex	例数 No. cases	发病率 Incidence rate（1/10⁵）	中标率 ASR China （1/10⁵）	世标率 ASR World （1/10⁵）	累积率 Cumulative rate（0~74，%）
全市 All areas	合计 Both	50 070	367.88	200.42	192.12	21.27
	男性 Male	24 752	364.46	188.94	184.92	21.31
	女性 Female	25 318	371.30	214.10	201.32	21.45
城区 Urban areas	合计 Both	32 997	390.95	205.63	196.71	21.79
	男性 Male	16 113	382.76	189.81	185.47	21.29
	女性 Female	16 884	399.10	223.46	209.72	22.46
郊区 Peri-urban areas	合计 Both	17 073	330.23	192.15	184.87	20.46
	男性 Male	8 639	334.61	188.25	184.92	21.35
	女性 Female	8 434	325.86	198.72	187.46	19.85

4.2.2 北京市全部恶性肿瘤年龄别发病率

2017 年北京市全部恶性肿瘤的年龄别发病率在 0~19 岁时处于较低水平，自 20~24 岁年龄组开始快速上升，在 80~84 岁年龄组达到高峰。15~59 岁年龄组女性年龄别发病率始终高于男性，自 60~64 岁年龄组起男性发病率高于女性。城区和郊区恶性肿瘤年龄别发病率变化趋势基本相同。30 岁以下城区和郊区各年龄组发病率差别不大，30 岁以上各年龄组除 85 岁及以上年龄组外，城区各年龄组发病率均高于郊区（表 4.2.2，图 4.2.1 至图 4.2.3）。

4.2.2 Age-specific incidence rate for all cancer sites in Beijing

Age-specific incidence rate was relatively low at the age group of 0-19 years, and increased sharply from the age group of 20-24 years, which peaked at the age group of 80-84 years. Age-specific incidence rate for age group of 15-59 years were consistently higher in females than that in males, and since then the age-specific incidence rate for males exceeded that for females. The overall trends of age-specific incidence rate in urban areas was similar to that in peri-areas. The age-specific incidence rates were similar in urban and peri-urban areas for people below 30 years of age; the age-specific incidence rates were higher in urban areas than that in peri-urban areas in people above 30 years old, except in the age group of 85 years and above (Table 4.2.2, Figure 4.2.1-4.2.3).

表 4.2.2 2017 年北京市户籍居民恶性肿瘤年龄别发病率 (1/10^5)

Table 4.2.2 Age-specific incidence rate of all cancer sites in Beijing, 2017 (1/10^5)

年龄组 Age group (years)	全市 All areas			城区 Urban areas			郊区 Peri-urban areas		
	合计 Both	男性 Male	女性 Female	合计 Both	男性 Male	女性 Female	合计 Both	男性 Male	女性 Female
合计 Total	367.88	364.46	371.30	390.95	382.76	399.10	330.23	334.61	325.86
0~	26.31	32.75	19.42	26.37	37.72	14.24	26.23	26.77	25.65
1~	16.75	18.96	14.39	18.46	21.53	15.18	14.05	14.90	13.16
5~	9.32	10.22	8.37	9.57	9.25	9.91	8.92	11.83	5.81
10~	11.22	12.42	9.94	11.86	12.35	11.33	10.31	12.53	7.97
15~	14.62	14.26	14.99	12.54	9.10	16.01	17.87	22.21	13.35
20~	32.62	21.70	43.47	32.20	23.90	40.28	33.41	17.68	49.68
25~	68.75	47.41	90.73	70.13	52.17	88.73	66.80	40.68	93.53
30~	98.99	63.05	135.22	109.84	67.76	152.20	82.93	56.10	110.05
35~	135.78	86.17	186.08	141.46	89.31	193.73	125.79	80.75	172.43
40~	201.55	111.60	293.74	208.56	121.45	297.91	190.46	95.97	287.16
45~	274.73	179.25	370.96	282.41	179.23	385.52	264.06	179.29	350.52
50~	374.17	301.99	448.82	387.80	308.31	472.15	354.77	292.71	416.66
55~	482.94	460.00	506.17	491.00	465.51	517.09	468.87	450.22	487.40
60~	648.93	688.89	610.93	662.69	685.58	640.83	624.90	694.71	559.03
65~	810.45	934.51	693.39	827.91	925.19	734.41	781.97	950.10	628.01
70~	1 071.83	1 309.48	861.19	1 089.06	1 284.43	916.92	1 044.77	1 348.50	773.04
75~	1 298.31	1 577.67	1 067.27	1 310.50	1 562.11	1 110.76	1 271.38	1 609.71	965.22
80~	1 405.99	1 718.03	1 127.63	1 422.20	1 705.27	1 170.14	1 360.54	1 753.67	1 008.09
85+	1 221.32	1 462.61	1 007.92	1 210.61	1 408.38	1 027.30	1 258.59	1 674.20	946.71

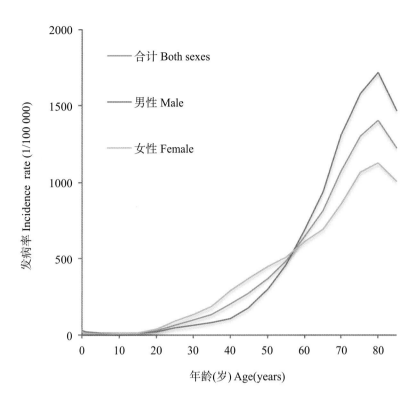

图 4.2.1 2017 年北京市户籍居民恶性肿瘤年龄别发病率
Figure 4.2.1 Age-specific incidence rate of all cancer sites in Beijing, 2017

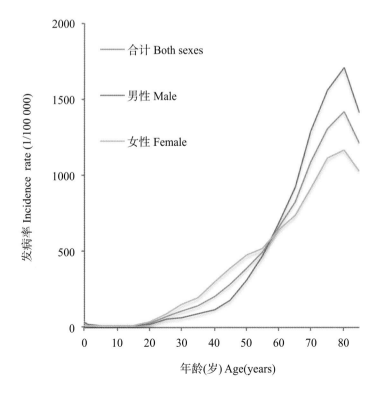

图 4.2.2 2017 年北京市城区户籍居民恶性肿瘤年龄别发病率
Figure 4.2.2 Age-specific incidence rate of all cancer sites in urban areas of Beijing, 2017

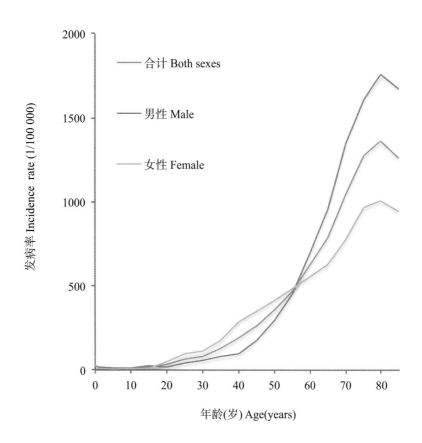

图 4.2.3 2017 年北京市郊区户籍居民恶性肿瘤年龄别发病率
Figure 4.2.3 Age-specific incidence rate of all cancer sites in peri-urban areas of Beijing, 2017

4.2.3 北京市全部恶性肿瘤死亡情况

2017年，北京市恶性肿瘤死亡报告26047例（男性15500例，女性10547例），其中城区16986例，占65.21%，郊区9061例，占34.79%。北京市2017年恶性肿瘤死亡率为191.38/10万（男性228.23/10万，女性154.68/10万），中标死亡率为81.39/10万，世标死亡率为80.51/10万，0~74岁累积死亡率为8.62%。城区死亡率为201.25/10万（男性237.12/10万，女性165.56/10万），中标死亡率为77.95/10万，世标死亡率为77.36/10万，0~74岁累积死亡率为8.21%。郊区死亡率为175.26/10万（男性213.72/10万，女性136.89/10万），中标

4.2.3 Mortality of all cancer sites in Beijing

In 2017, there were 26,047 cancer deaths (15,500 for males and 10,547 for females) in Beijing, with 16,986 deaths(65.21%) in the urban areas and 9,061 deaths (34.79%) in the peri-urban areas. The mortality rate of all cancer sites was 191.38 per 100,000 in 2017 (228.23 for males and 154.68 for females), with an ASR China of 81.39 per 100,000, an ASR World of 80.51 per 100,000, and a cumulative mortality rate for subjects aged 0 to 74 years of 8.62%. The mortality rate of all cancers in the urban areas was 201.25 per 100,000 (237.12 per 100,000 for males and 165.56 per 100,000 for females), with an ASR China of 77.95 per 100,000, an ASR World of 77.36 per 100,000, and a cumulative rate for subjects aged 0 to 74 years of 8.21%. The mortality rate of all

死亡率为87.45/10万，世标死亡率为85.97/10万，0~74岁累积死亡率为9.28%。城区和郊区相比，城区男性和女性死亡率均高于郊区，但城区男性和女性的中标死亡率、世标死亡率和0~74岁累积死亡率均低于郊区（表4.2.3）。

北京市全部恶性肿瘤世标死亡率由2008年的85.40/10万下降到2017年的80.51/10万，年均变化百分比为-1.06%（P=0.005）；男性和女性死亡10年间年均变化百分比分别为-1.01%（P=0.007）和-1.14%（P=0.006）。

cancer sites in the peri-urban areas was 175.26 per 100,000 (213.72 for males and 136.89 for females), with an ASR China of 87.45 per 100,000, an ASR World of 85.97 per 100,000, and a cumulative rate for subjects aged 0 to 74 years of 9.28%. The crude mortality rates of all cancer sites were higher in the urban areas than those in the peri-urban areas for both sexes. The ASR China and ASR World for mortality and the cumulative mortality rate were lower in urban areas than those in peri-urban areas (Table 4.2.3).

The ASR World for mortality of all cancers in Beijing decreased from 85.40 per 100,000 in 2008 to 80.51 per 100,000 in 2017, with an APC of -1.06% (P=0.005) during the period of time. And the APCs in the last 10 years for males and females were -1.01% (P=0.007) and -1.14% (P=0.006), respectively.

表4.2.3 2017年北京市户籍居民全部恶性肿瘤死亡情况
Table 4.2.3 Mortality of all cancer sites in Beijing, 2017

地区 Areas	性别 Sex	例数 No. deaths	死亡率 Mortality rate （1/10^5）	中标率 ASR China （1/10^5）	世标率 ASR World （1/10^5）	累积率 Cumulative rate(0~74,%)
全市 All areas	合计 Both	26 047	191.38	81.39	80.51	8.62
	男性 Male	15 500	228.23	100.52	99.94	10.98
	女性 Female	10 547	154.68	63.83	62.58	6.41
城区 Urban areas	合计 Both	16 986	201.25	77.95	77.36	8.21
	男性 Male	9 982	237.12	94.55	94.35	10.23
	女性 Female	7 004	165.56	62.72	61.62	6.31
郊区 Peri-urban areas	合计 Both	9 061	175.26	87.45	85.97	9.28
	男性 Male	5 518	213.72	110.87	109.62	12.18
	女性 Female	3 543	136.89	65.95	64.34	6.60

4.2.4 北京市全部恶性肿瘤年龄别死亡率

北京市恶性肿瘤年龄别死亡率在 40~44 岁年龄组以前处于较低水平，自 40~44 岁年龄组开始年龄别死亡率快速上升，在 85 岁及以上年龄组达到高峰；自 45~49 岁年龄组开始，男性各年龄别死亡率始终高于女性。城区和郊区年龄别死亡率的变化趋势基本相同。30 岁以下城区和郊区各年龄组死亡率差别不大，30 岁以上各年龄组除 85 岁及以上年龄组外，郊区各年龄别死亡率均高于城区（表 4.2.4，图 4.2.4 至图 4.2.6）。

4.2.4 Age-specific mortality rate for all cancer sites in Beijing

Age-specific mortality rate was relatively low before 40 years old, and increased dramatically since then, which peaked at the age group of 85 years and above. Age-specific mortality rate for males was consistently higher in males than that in females since the age group of 45-49 years. The overall trend of age-specific mortality rate in urban areas was similar to that in peri-urban areas. The age-specific mortality rates were similar in urban and peri-urban areas in people below 30 years old, but higher in peri-urban areas above 30 years old, except in the age group of 85 years and above (Table 4.2.4, Figure 4.2.4-4.2.6).

表 4.2.4　2017 年北京市户籍居民恶性肿瘤年龄别死亡率（1/10^5）
Table 4.2.4 Age-specific mortality rate of all cancer sites in Beijing, 2017(1/10^5)

年龄组 Age groups	全市 All areas			城区 Urban areas			郊区 Peri-urban areas		
	合计 Both	男性 Male	女性 Female	合计 Both	男性 Male	女性 Female	合计 Both	男性 Male	女性 Female
合计 Total	191.38	228.23	154.68	201.25	237.12	165.56	175.26	213.72	136.89
0~	6.89	6.07	7.77	6.88	6.66	7.12	6.90	5.35	8.55
1~	2.49	2.57	2.40	2.99	3.15	2.81	1.70	1.66	1.75
5~	2.29	2.38	2.18	2.53	2.72	2.33	1.88	1.82	1.94
10~	3.21	2.59	3.86	3.65	1.76	5.67	2.58	3.76	1.33
15~	3.48	4.14	2.81	3.80	3.03	4.57	2.98	5.84	0.00
25~	4.33	4.56	4.09	4.14	4.74	3.51	4.60	4.31	4.90
30~	9.50	8.35	10.65	8.75	7.72	9.78	10.60	9.28	11.94
35~	16.96	15.45	18.49	13.82	10.87	16.78	22.47	23.36	21.55
40~	34.72	30.78	38.76	33.76	27.97	39.69	36.25	35.23	37.29
45~	62.54	68.28	56.76	57.97	61.65	54.30	68.89	77.40	60.20

续表

年龄组 Age groups	全市 All areas			城区 Urban areas			郊区 Peri-urban areas		
	合计 Both	男性 Male	女性 Female	合计 Both	男性 Male	女性 Female	合计 Both	男性 Male	女性 Female
55~	170.70	215.55	125.30	166.83	213.28	119.31	177.46	219.57	135.61
60~	259.88	347.66	176.40	246.52	331.41	165.44	283.20	376.22	195.42
65~	396.73	526.08	274.66	381.27	498.18	268.90	421.94	572.75	283.84
70~	638.82	826.85	472.16	601.61	748.38	472.29	697.25	949.08	471.95
75~	951.19	1 182.85	759.58	896.55	1 111.74	725.71	1 071.93	1 329.27	839.07
80~	1 334.56	1 647.96	1 054.99	1 314.95	1 610.94	1 051.39	1 389.53	1 751.40	1 065.11
85+	1 490.28	1 783.95	1 230.56	1 496.75	1 767.34	1 245.96	1 467.79	1 848.77	1 181.90

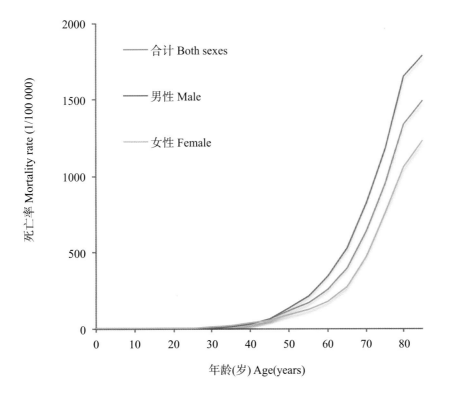

图 4.2.4 2017 年北京市户籍居民恶性肿瘤年龄别死亡率

Figure 4.2.4 Age-specific mortality rate of all cancer sites in Beijing, 2017

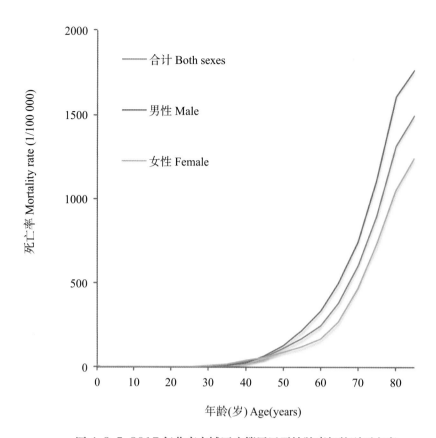

图 4.2.5　2017 年北京市城区户籍居民恶性肿瘤年龄别死亡率

Figure 4.2.5 Age-specific mortality rate of all cancer sites in urban areas of Beijing, 2017

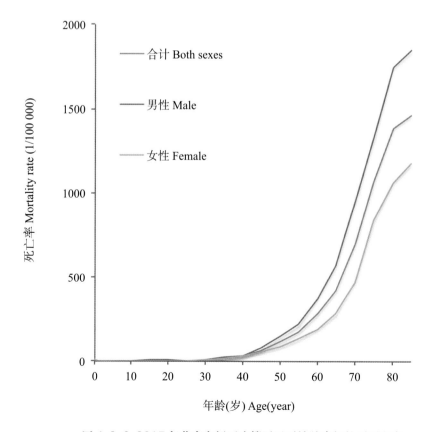

图 4.2.6　2017 年北京市郊区户籍居民恶性肿瘤年龄别死亡率

Figure 4.2.6 Age-specific mortality rate of all cancer sites in peri-urban areas of Beijing, 2017

4.2.5 北京市全部恶性肿瘤地区分布

2017 年，北京市 16 个辖区恶性肿瘤世标发病率和死亡率呈现明显的差异，城区世标发病率高于郊区，郊区世标死亡率高于城区（图 4.2.7 至图 4.2.8）。

4.2.5 Incidence and mortality rates of all cancer sites by district of Beijing

In 2017, there were significant differences among the 16 districts in ASR World incidence and mortality of all cancers in Beijing. The incidence rate was higher in urban areas than that in peri-urban areas, while the mortality rate was higher in peri-urban areas than that in urban areas (Figure 4.2.7-4.2.8).

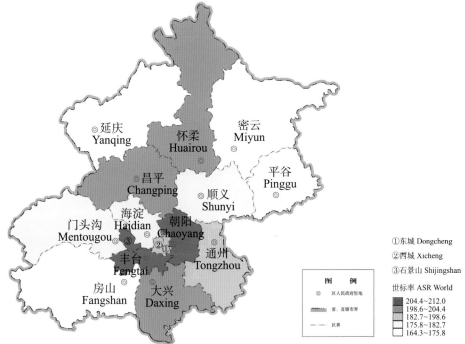

图 4.2.7 2017 年北京市户籍居民全部恶性肿瘤发病率（1/10^5）地区分布情况

Figure 4.2.7 Incidence rates of all cancer sites by district in Beijing, 2017 (1/10^5)

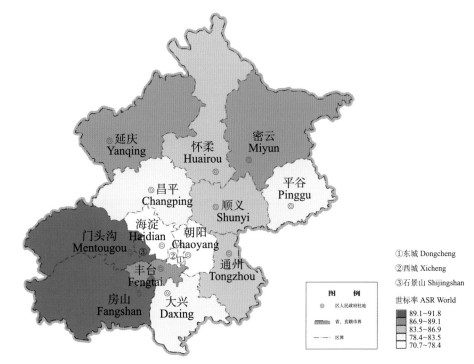

图 4.2.8 2017 年北京市户籍居民全部恶性肿瘤死亡率（1/10^5）地区分布情况

Figure 4.2.8 Mortality rates of all cancer sites by district in Beijing, 2017 (1/10^5)

4.3 北京市前 10 位恶性肿瘤发病与死亡

4.3.1 北京市前 10 位恶性肿瘤发病情况

2017 年，北京市男性恶性肿瘤发病第 1 位的是肺癌，其次为结直肠癌、肝癌、胃癌和前列腺癌。女性恶性肿瘤发病第 1 位的是乳腺癌，其次为肺癌、甲状腺癌、结直肠癌和子宫体癌（表 4.3.1，图 4.3.1 至图 4.3.4）。

4.3 The top 10 cancer sites in Beijing in terms of incidence and mortality

4.3.1 Top 10 cancer sites in Beijing in terms of incidence

In 2017, the most common cancer for males was lung cancer, followed by colorectal, liver, stomach and prostate cancers. The most common cancer for females was breast cancer, followed by lung, thyroid, colorectal, and uterus cancers (Table 4.3.1, Figure 4.3.1-4.3.4).

表 4.3.1　2017 年北京市户籍居民恶性肿瘤发病前 10 位
Table 4.3.1 Top 10 cancer sites in terms of incidence in Beijing, 2017

顺位 Rank	部位 Sites	男性 Male				
		例数 No. cases	构成比 Freq.(%)	粗率 Crude rate （1/10^5）	中标率 ASR China （1/10^5）	世标率 ASR World （1/10^5）
1	肺 Lung	6 041	24.41	88.95	41.67	41.60
2	结直肠 Colon-rectum	3 620	14.63	53.30	25.74	25.55
3	肝 Liver	1 670	6.75	24.59	12.55	12.54
4	胃 Stomach	1 667	6.73	24.55	11.65	11.52
5	前列腺 Prostate	1 606	6.49	23.65	10.50	10.30
6	肾 Kidney	1 272	5.14	18.73	10.32	10.03
7	膀胱 Bladder	1 257	5.08	18.51	8.51	8.44
8	甲状腺 Thyroid	1 209	4.88	17.80	16.73	13.66
9	食管 Esophagus	964	3.89	14.19	6.47	6.61
10	淋巴瘤 Lymphoma	814	3.29	11.99	6.82	6.56

	女性 Female				
部位 Sites	例数 No. cases	构成比 Freq.(%)	粗率 Crude rate (1/10⁵)	中标率 ASR China (1/10⁵)	世标率 ASR World (1/10⁵)
乳腺 Breast	5 119	20.22	75.07	46.27	43.45
肺 Lung	4 084	16.13	59.89	27.38	26.95
甲状腺 Thyroid	3 463	13.68	50.79	44.93	37.95
结直肠 Colon-rectum	2 634	10.40	38.63	17.28	16.91
子宫体 Uterus	1 358	5.36	19.92	11.77	11.43
卵巢 Ovary	842	3.33	12.35	7.57	7.26
肾 Kidney	820	3.24	12.03	5.80	5.74
胃 Stomach	804	3.18	11.79	5.62	5.37
肝 Liver	694	2.74	10.18	4.32	4.31
子宫颈 Cervix	652	2.58	9.56	6.92	6.17

发病率 Incidence rate(1/100 000)

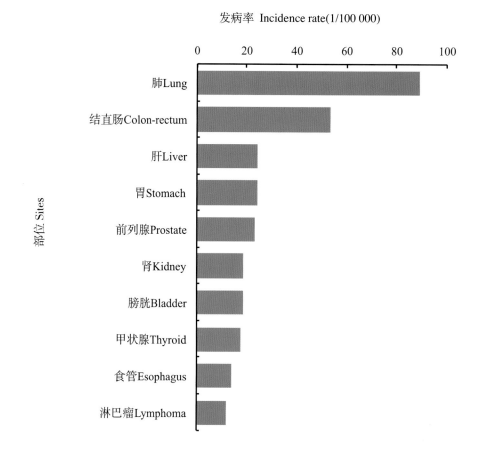

图 4.3.1 2017 年北京市户籍居民男性恶性肿瘤发病率前 10 位
Figure 4.3.1 Top 10 cancer sites for males in terms of incidence in Beijing, 2017

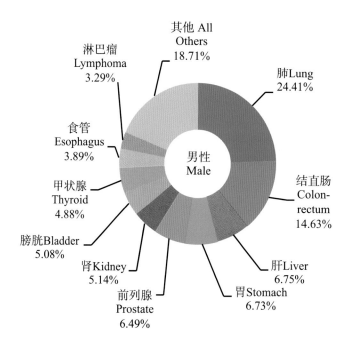

图 4.3.2 2017 年北京市户籍居民男性恶性肿瘤发病构成前 10 位
Figure 4.3.2 Distribution of the top 10 new cancer cases by site for males in Beijing, 2017

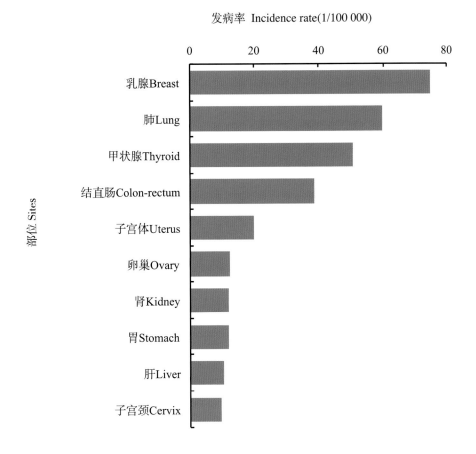

图 4.3.3 2017 年北京市户籍居民女性恶性肿瘤发病率前 10 位
Figure 4.3.3 Top 10 cancer sites for females in terms of incidence in Beijing, 2017

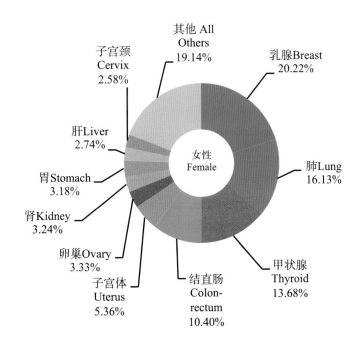

图 4.3.4 2017 年北京市户籍居民女性恶性肿瘤发病构成前 10 位
Figure 4.3.4 Distribution of the top 10 new cancer cases by site for females in Beijing, 2017

4.3.2 北京市前 10 位恶性肿瘤死亡情况

2017 年，北京市不论男性和女性，恶性肿瘤死亡第 1 位的均为肺癌，其次为结直肠癌。男性恶性肿瘤死亡第 3 ~ 5 位的分别为肝癌、胃癌和食管癌，女性分别为乳腺癌、肝癌和胰腺癌（表 4.3.2，图 4.3.5 至图 4.3.8）。

4.3.2 Top 10 cancer sites in terms of mortality in Beijing

For both sexes, lung cancer was the leading cause of cancer deaths, followed by colorectal cancer. As for males, liver cancer, stomach cancer, and esophagus cancer were the 3rd, 4th, and 5th leading causes of deaths in all cancers, respectively. And for females, breast cancer, liver cancer, and pancreas cancer were the 3rd, 4th, and 5th leading causes of cancer deaths, respectively (Table 4.3.2, Figure 4.3.5-4.3.8).

表 4.3.2　2017 年北京市户籍居民恶性肿瘤死亡前 10 位
Table 4.3.2 Top 10 cancer sites in terms of mortality in Beijing, 2017

顺位 Rank	部位 Sites	男性 Male				
		例数 No. deaths	构成比 Freq.(%)	粗率 Crude rate （1/10^5）	中标率 ASR China （1/10^5）	世标率 ASR World （1/10^5）
1	肺 Lung	4 850	31.29	71.41	30.99	30.89
2	结直肠 Colon-rectum	1 692	10.92	24.91	10.28	10.19
3	肝 Liver	1 614	10.41	23.77	11.63	11.60
4	胃 Stomach	1 163	7.50	17.12	7.29	7.14
5	食管 Esophagus	856	5.52	12.60	5.48	5.57
6	胰腺 Pancreas	766	4.94	11.28	5.27	5.18
7	前列腺 Prostate	613	3.95	9.03	3.06	3.03
8	白血病 Leukemia	527	3.40	7.76	4.04	3.96
9	膀胱 Bladder	524	3.38	7.72	2.64	2.69
10	淋巴瘤 Lymphoma	522	3.37	7.69	3.49	3.39

	女性 Female				
部位 Sites	例数 No. deaths	构成比 Freq.(%)	粗率 Crude rate ($1/10^5$)	中标率 ASR China ($1/10^5$)	世标率 ASR World ($1/10^5$)
肺 Lung	2 540	24.08	37.25	14.16	13.84
结直肠 Colon-rectum	1 290	12.23	18.92	6.83	6.74
乳腺 Breast	1 067	10.12	15.65	7.40	7.29
肝 Liver	635	6.02	9.31	3.63	3.58
胰腺 Pancreas	554	5.25	8.12	3.12	3.08
胃 Stomach	552	5.23	8.10	3.57	3.41
卵巢 Ovary	473	4.48	6.94	3.44	3.38
淋巴瘤 Lymphoma	407	3.86	5.97	2.53	2.50
胆囊 Gallbladder	394	3.74	5.78	2.21	2.14
白血病 Leukemia	340	3.22	4.99	2.60	2.58

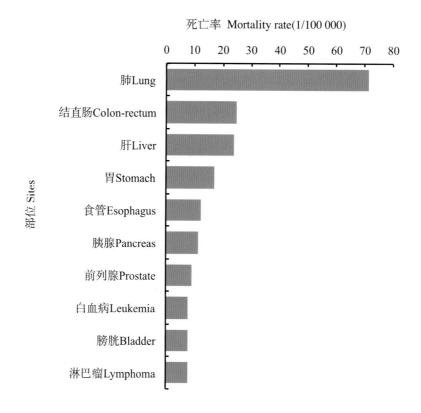

图 4.3.5　2017 年北京市户籍居民男性恶性肿瘤死亡率前 10 位
Figure 4.3.5 Top 10 cancer sites in terms of mortality for males in Beijing, 2017

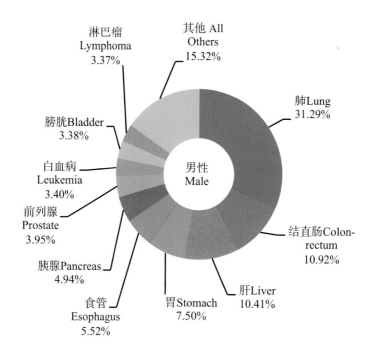

图 4.3.6　2017 年北京市户籍居民男性恶性肿瘤死亡构成前 10 位
Figure 4.3.6 Distribution of the top 10 cancer sites in terms of mortality for males in Beijing, 2017

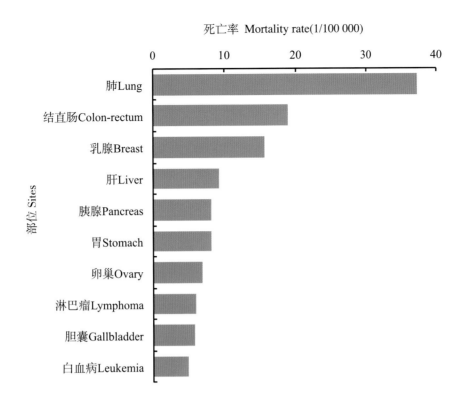

图 4.3.7 2017 年北京市户籍居民女性恶性肿瘤死亡率前 10 位

Figure 4.3.7 Top 10 cancer sites in terms of mortality for females in Beijing, 2017

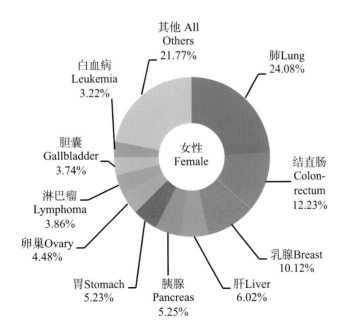

图 4.3.8 2017 年北京市户籍居民女性恶性肿瘤死亡构成前 10 位

Figure 4.3.8 Distribution of the top 10 cancer sites in terms of mortality for females in Beijing, 2017

4.3.3 北京市城区前 10 位恶性肿瘤发病情况

2017 年北京市城区男性恶性肿瘤发病第 1 位的是肺癌，其次为结直肠癌、前列腺癌、胃癌和肝癌。城区女性发病第 1 位的是乳腺癌，其次为肺癌、甲状腺癌、结直肠癌和子宫体癌（表 4.3.3，图 4.3.9 至图 4.3.12）。

4.3.3 Top 10 cancer sites in terms of incidence in urban areas of Beijing

The most common cancer for males was lung cancer in urban areas of Beijing in 2017, followed by colorectal cancer, prostate cancer, stomach cancer, and liver cancer. And the most common cancer for females was breast cancer, followed by lung cancer, thyroid cancer, colorectal cancer, and uterus cancer (Table 4.3.3, Figure 4.3.9–4.3.12).

表 4.3.3　2017 年北京市城区户籍居民恶性肿瘤发病前 10 位
Table 4.3.3 Top 10 cancer sites in terms of incidence in urban areas of Beijing, 2017

顺位 Rank	部位 Sites	男性 Male				
		例数 No. cases	构成比 Freq.(%)	粗率 Crude rate （1/10⁵）	中标率 ASR China （1/10⁵）	世标率 ASR World （1/10⁵）
1	肺 Lung	3 718	23.07	88.32	38.98	38.91
2	结直肠 Colon-rectum	2 519	15.63	59.84	27.47	27.27
3	前列腺 Prostate	1 187	7.37	28.20	11.94	11.72
4	胃 Stomach	1 122	6.96	26.65	11.86	11.72
5	肝 Liver	1 021	6.34	24.25	11.60	11.64
6	肾 Kidney	889	5.52	21.12	11.28	10.95
7	膀胱 Bladder	865	5.37	20.55	8.85	8.75
8	甲状腺 Thyroid	818	5.08	19.43	18.74	15.19
9	胰腺 Pancreas	532	3.30	12.64	5.76	5.70
10	淋巴瘤 Lymphoma	530	3.29	12.59	6.87	6.61

女性 Female					
部位 Sites	例数 No. cases	构成比 Freq.(%)	粗率 Crude rate ($1/10^5$)	中标率 ASR China ($1/10^5$)	世标率 ASR World ($1/10^5$)
乳腺 Breast	3 468	20.54	81.97	49.50	46.65
肺 Lung	2 730	16.17	64.53	28.29	27.83
甲状腺 Thyroid	2 256	13.36	53.33	48.07	40.25
结直肠 Colon-rectum	1 818	10.77	42.97	18.16	17.75
子宫体 Uterus	853	5.05	20.16	11.73	11.44
胃 Stomach	579	3.43	13.69	6.18	5.93
肾 Kidney	556	3.29	13.14	6.03	5.94
卵巢 Ovary	544	3.22	12.86	7.85	7.49
淋巴瘤 Lymphoma	453	2.68	10.71	5.58	5.32
肝 Liver	446	2.64	10.54	4.03	4.07

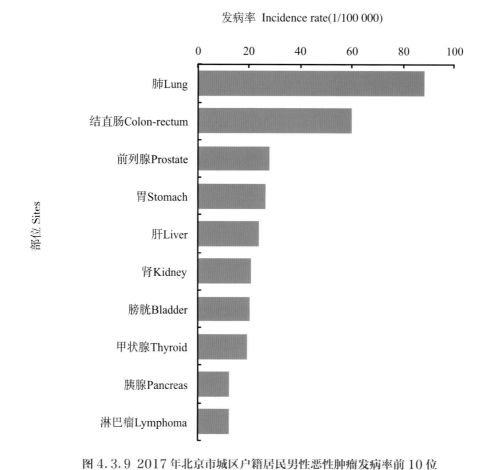

图 4.3.9 2017 年北京市城区户籍居民男性恶性肿瘤发病率前 10 位
Figure 4.3.9 Top 10 cancer sites in terms of incidence for males in urban areas of Beijing, 2017

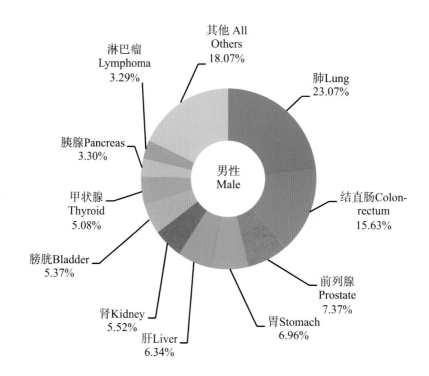

图 4.3.10 2017 年北京市城区户籍居民男性恶性肿瘤发病构成前 10 位
Figure 4.3.10 Distribution of the top 10 cancer sites in terms of incidence for males in urban areas of Beijing, 2017

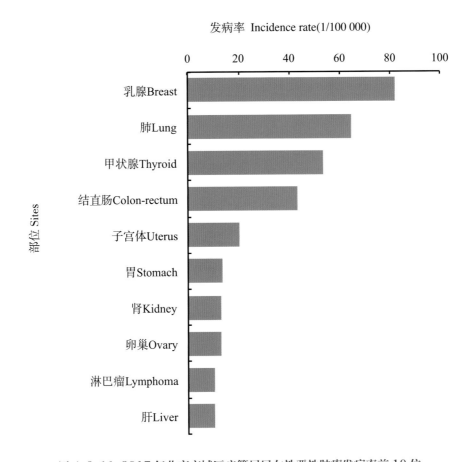

图 4.3.11　2017 年北京市城区户籍居民女性恶性肿瘤发病率前 10 位
Figure 4.3.11 Top 10 cancer sites in terms of incidence for females in urban areas of Beijing, 2017

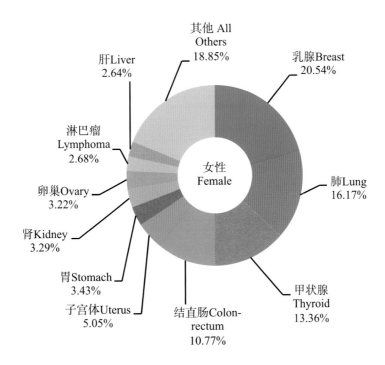

图 4.3.12　2017 年北京市城区户籍居民女性恶性肿瘤发病构成前 10 位
Figure 4.3.12 Distribution of the top 10 cancer sites in terms of incidence for females in urban areas of Beijing, 2017

4.3.4 北京市城区前 10 位恶性肿瘤死亡情况

2017 年，北京市城区不论男性和女性，恶性肿瘤死亡第 1 位的均为肺癌，其次为结直肠癌。男性恶性肿瘤死亡第 3 ~ 5 位的分别为肝癌、胃癌和胰腺癌，女性分别为乳腺癌、肝癌和胰腺癌（表 4.3.4，图 4.3.13 至图 4.3.16）。

4.3.4 Top 10 cancer sites in terms of mortality in urban areas of Beijing

For both sexes, lung cancer was the leading cause of cancer deaths in urban areas of Beijing in 2017, followed by colorectal cancer. Liver cancer, stomach cancer and pancreas cancer were the 3rd, 4th, and 5th leading causes of cancer deaths in all cancers, respectively, for males. And for females, breast cancer, liver cancer and pancreas cancer were the 3rd, 4th, and 5th leading causes of cancer deaths in all cancers, respectively (Table 4.3.4, Figure 4.3.13-4.3.16).

表 4.3.4 2017 年北京市城区户籍居民恶性肿瘤死亡前 10 位
Table 4.3.4 Top 10 cancer sites in terms of mortality in urban areas of Beijing, 2017

顺位 Rank	部位 Sites	男性 Male				
		例数 No. deaths	构成比 Freq.(%)	粗率 Crude rate （1/10^5）	中标率 ASR China （1/10^5）	世标率 ASR World （1/10^5）
1	肺 Lung	3 013	30.18	71.57	28.03	28.08
2	结直肠 Colon-rectum	1 219	12.21	28.96	10.89	10.77
3	肝 Liver	977	9.79	23.21	10.54	10.50
4	胃 Stomach	768	7.69	18.24	7.04	6.91
5	胰腺 Pancreas	521	5.22	12.38	5.40	5.36
6	食管 Esophagus	462	4.63	10.97	4.45	4.58
7	前列腺 Prostate	455	4.56	10.81	3.20	3.15
8	膀胱 Bladder	356	3.57	8.46	2.42	2.51
9	淋巴瘤 Lymphoma	341	3.42	8.10	3.33	3.24
10	白血病 Leukemia	338	3.39	8.03	3.64	3.63

女性 Female					
部位 Sites	例数 No. deaths	构成比 Freq.(%)	粗率 Crude rate （1/10^5）	中标率 ASR China （1/10^5）	世标率 ASR World （1/10^5）
肺 Lung	1 589	22.69	37.56	12.86	12.52
结直肠 Colon-rectum	892	12.74	21.08	6.79	6.76
乳腺 Breast	745	10.64	17.61	7.90	7.82
肝 Liver	400	5.71	9.46	3.17	3.16
胰腺 Pancreas	396	5.65	9.36	3.26	3.24
胃 Stomach	387	5.53	9.15	3.68	3.56
卵巢 Ovary	318	4.54	7.52	3.59	3.54
淋巴瘤 Lymphoma	277	3.95	6.55	2.59	2.53
胆囊 Gallbladder	238	3.40	5.63	1.90	1.82
肾 Kidney	230	3.28	5.44	1.59	1.59

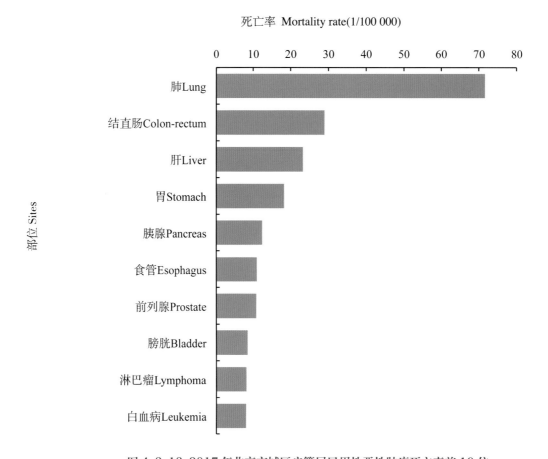

图 4.3.13 2017 年北京市城区户籍居民男性恶性肿瘤死亡率前 10 位

Figure 4.3.13 Top 10 cancer sites in terms of mortality for males in urban areas of Beijing, 2017

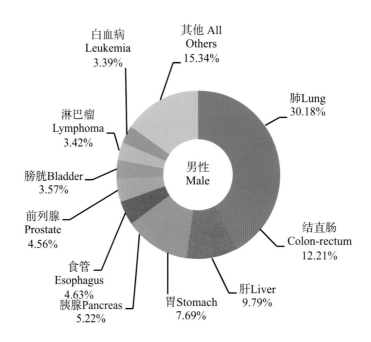

图 4.3.14 2017 年北京市城区户籍居民男性恶性肿瘤死亡构成前 10 位

Figure 4.3.14 Distribution of the top 10 cancer sites in terms of mortality for males in urban areas of Beijing, 2017

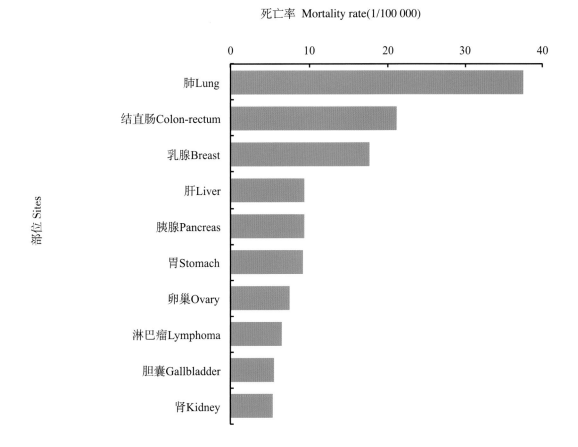

图 4.3.15 2017 年北京市城区户籍居民女性恶性肿瘤死亡率前 10 位

Figure 4.3.15 Top 10 cancer sites in terms of mortality for females in urban areas of Beijing, 2017

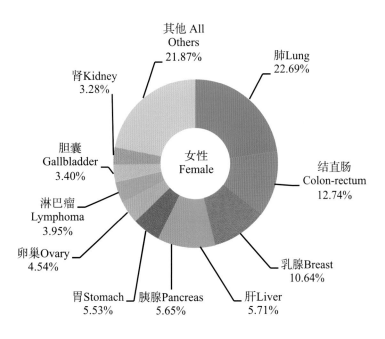

图 4.3.16 2017 年北京市城区户籍居民女性恶性肿瘤死亡构成前 10 位

Figure 4.3.16 Distribution of the top 10 cancer sites in terms of mortality for females in urban areas of Beijing, 2017

4.3.5 北京市郊区前 10 位恶性肿瘤发病情况

2017 年北京市郊区男性恶性肿瘤发病第 1 位的是肺癌，其次为结直肠癌、肝癌、胃癌和食管癌。郊区女性发病第 1 位的是乳腺癌，其次为肺癌、甲状腺癌、结直肠癌和子宫体癌（表 4.3.5，图 4.3.17 至图 4.3.20）。

4.3.5 Top 10 cancer sites in terms of incidence in peri-urban areas of Beijing

The most common cancer for males was lung cancer in peri-urban areas of Beijing in 2017, followed by colorectal cancer, liver cancer, stomach cancer, and esophagus cancer. And the most common cancer for females was breast cancer, followed by lung cancer, thyroid cancer, colorectal cancer, and uterus cancer (Table 4.3.5, Figure 4.3.17-4.3.20).

表 4.3.5　2017 年北京市郊区户籍居民恶性肿瘤发病前 10 位
Table 4.3.5 Top 10 cancer sites in terms of incidence in peri-urban areas of Beijing, 2017

顺位 Rank	部位 Sites	男性 Male				
		例数 No. cases	构成比 Freq.(%)	粗率 Crude rate （1/10^5）	中标率 ASR China （1/10^5）	世标率 ASR World （1/10^5）
1	肺 Lung	2 323	26.89	89.97	46.57	46.45
2	结直肠 Colon-rectum	1 101	12.74	42.64	22.66	22.52
3	肝 Liver	649	7.51	25.14	14.03	14.01
4	胃 Stomach	545	6.31	21.11	11.26	11.18
5	食管 Esophagus	445	5.15	17.24	8.64	8.77
6	前列腺 Prostate	419	4.85	16.23	8.06	7.97
7	膀胱 Bladder	392	4.54	15.18	7.92	7.89
8	甲状腺 Thyroid	391	4.53	15.14	13.64	11.33
9	肾 Kidney	383	4.43	14.83	8.70	8.46
10	淋巴瘤 Lymphoma	284	3.29	11.00	6.72	6.48

女性 Female					
部位 Sites	例数 No. cases	构成比 Freq.(%)	粗率 Crude rate （1/10^5）	中标率 ASR China （1/10^5）	世标率 ASR World （1/10^5）
乳腺 Breast	1 651	19.58	63.79	40.89	38.10
肺 Lung	1 354	16.05	52.31	25.99	25.63
甲状腺 Thyroid	1 207	14.31	46.63	40.07	34.44
结直肠 Colon-rectum	816	9.68	31.53	15.66	15.40
子宫体 Uterus	505	5.99	19.51	11.75	11.35
卵巢 Ovary	298	3.53	11.51	7.13	6.89
肾 Kidney	264	3.13	10.20	5.35	5.35
子宫颈 Cervix	261	3.09	10.08	7.51	6.59
肝 Liver	248	2.94	9.58	4.76	4.68
胃 Stomach	225	2.67	8.69	4.70	4.45

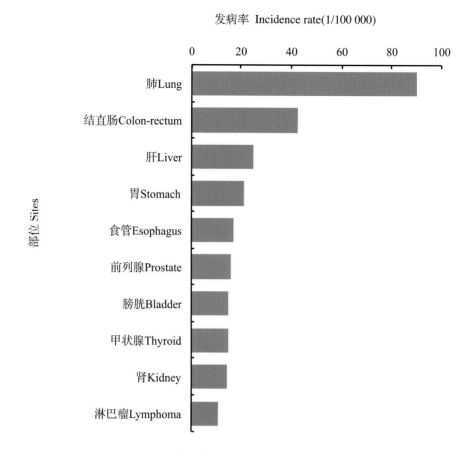

图 4.3.17 2017 年北京市郊区户籍居民男性恶性肿瘤发病率前 10 位
Figure 4.3.17 Top 10 cancer sites in terms of incidence for males in peri-urban areas of Beijing, 2017

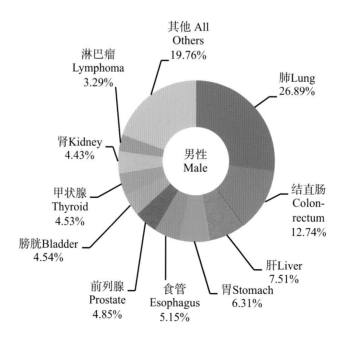

图 4.3.18 2017 年北京市郊区户籍居民男性恶性肿瘤发病构成前 10 位
Figure 4.3.18 Distribution of the top 10 cancer sites in terms of incidence for males in peri-urban areas of Beijing, 2017

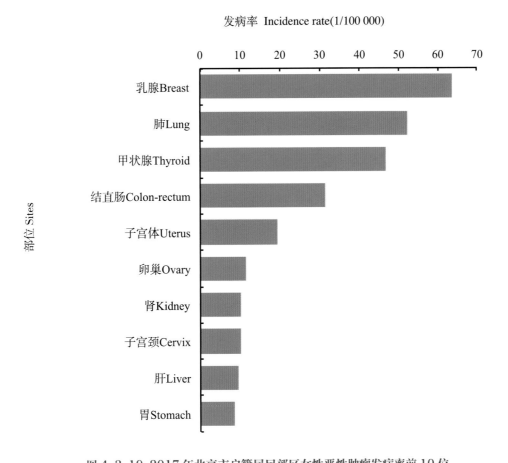

图 4.3.19 2017 年北京市户籍居民郊区女性恶性肿瘤发病率前 10 位

Figure 4.3.19 Top 10 cancer sites in terms of incidence for females in peri-urban areas of Beijing, 2017

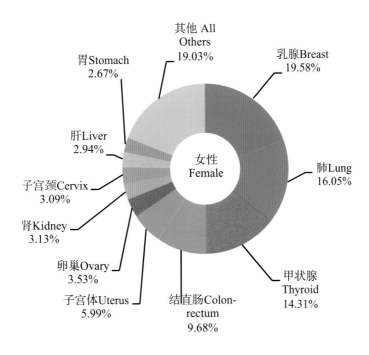

图 4.3.20 2017 年北京市户籍居民郊区女性恶性肿瘤发病构成前 10 位

Figure 4.3.20 Distribution of the top 10 cancer sites in terms of incidence for females in peri-urban areas of Beijing, 2017

4.3.6 北京市郊区前 10 位恶性肿瘤死亡情况

2017 年，北京市郊区不论男性和女性，死亡第 1 位的恶性肿瘤均为肺癌。男性恶性肿瘤死亡第 2 ~ 5 位的分别为肝癌、结直肠癌、胃癌和食管癌，女性分别为结直肠癌、乳腺癌、肝癌和胃癌（表4.3.6，图 4.3.21 至图 4.3.24 ）。

4.3.6 Top 10 cancer sites in terms of mortality in peri-urban areas of Beijing

For both sexes, lung cancer was the leading cause of cancer deaths in peri-urban areas of Beijing in 2017. As for males, liver cancer, colorectal cancer, stomach cancer, and esophagus cancer were the 2nd, 3rd, 4th, and 5th leading causes of cancer deaths in all kinds of cancers, respectively. And for females, colorectal cancer, breast cancer, liver cancer and stomach cancer were the 2nd, 3rd, 4th, and 5th leading causes of cancer deaths in all kinds of cancers, respectively (Table 4.3.6, Figure 4.3.21-4.3.24).

表 4.3.6   2017 年北京市郊区户籍居民恶性肿瘤死亡前 10 位
Table 4.3.6 Top 10 cancer sites in terms of mortality in peri-urban areas of Beijing, 2017

顺位 Rank	部位 Sites	例数 No. deaths	构成比 Freq.(%)	粗率 Crude rate (1/10^5)	中标率 ASR China (1/10^5)	世标率 ASR World (1/10^5)
	男性 Male					
1	肺 Lung	1 837	33.29	71.15	36.18	35.75
2	肝 Liver	637	11.54	24.67	13.38	13.42
3	结直肠 Colon-rectum	473	8.57	18.32	9.14	9.10
4	胃 Stomach	395	7.16	15.30	7.74	7.57
5	食管 Esophagus	394	7.14	15.26	7.55	7.61
6	胰腺 Pancreas	245	4.44	9.49	5.04	4.86
7	胆囊 Gallbladder	200	3.62	7.75	3.84	3.72
8	白血病 Leukemia	189	3.43	7.32	4.65	4.43
9	淋巴瘤 Lymphoma	181	3.28	7.01	3.77	3.66
10	膀胱 Bladder	168	3.04	6.51	3.04	3.03

	女性 Female				
部位 Sites	例数 No. deaths	构成比 Freq.(%)	粗率 Crude rate （1/10^5）	中标率 ASR China （1/10^5）	世标率 ASR World （1/10^5）
肺 Lung	951	26.84	36.74	16.59	16.31
结直肠 Colon-rectum	398	11.23	15.38	6.94	6.71
乳腺 Breast	322	9.09	12.44	6.59	6.39
肝 Liver	235	6.63	9.08	4.33	4.23
胃 Stomach	165	4.66	6.38	3.37	3.14
胰腺 Pancreas	158	4.46	6.10	2.83	2.75
胆囊 Gallbladder	156	4.40	6.03	2.76	2.73
卵巢 Ovary	155	4.37	5.99	3.16	3.11
淋巴瘤 Lymphoma	130	3.67	5.02	2.42	2.43
白血病 Leukemia	111	3.13	4.29	2.38	2.31

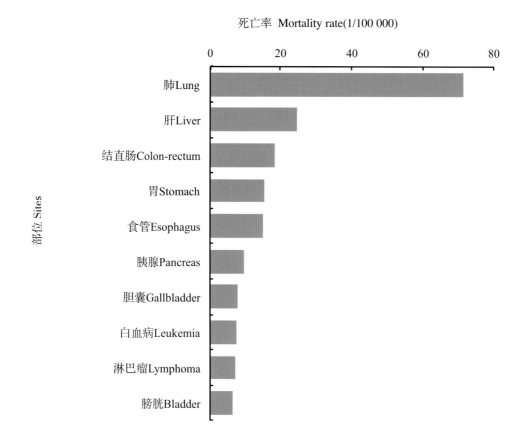

图 4.3.21 2017 年北京市郊区户籍居民男性恶性肿瘤死亡率前 10 位
Figure 4.3.21 Top 10 cancer sites in terms of mortality for males in peri-urban areas of Beijing, 2017

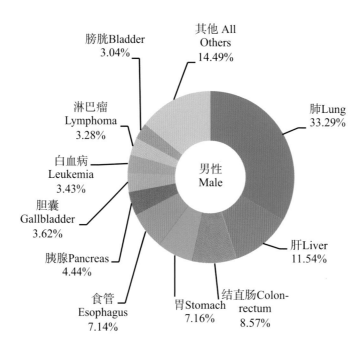

图 4.3.22 2017 年北京市郊区户籍居民男性恶性肿瘤死亡构成前 10 位
Figure 4.3.22 Distribution of the top 10 cancer sites in terms of mortality for males in peri-urban areas of Beijing, 2017

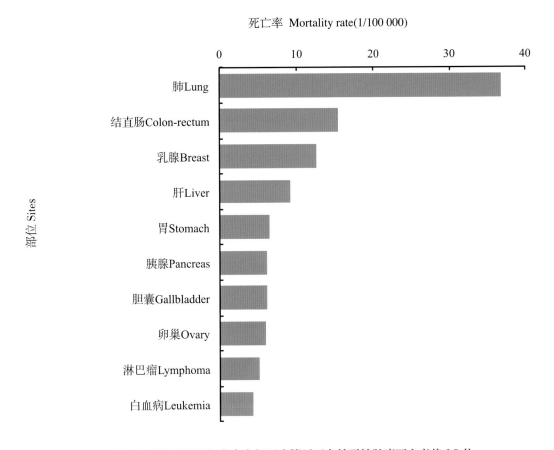

图 4.3.23 2017 年北京市郊区户籍居民女性恶性肿瘤死亡率前 10 位

Figure 4.3.23 Top 10 cancer sites in terms of mortality for females in peri-urban areas of Beijing, 2017

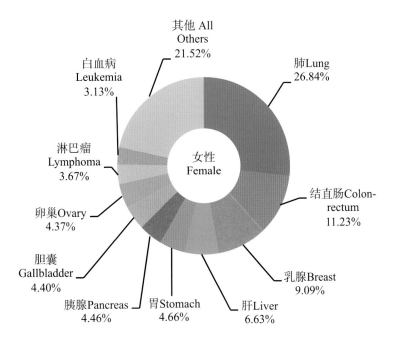

图 4.3.24 2017 年北京市郊区户籍居民女性恶性肿瘤死亡构成前 10 位

Figure 4.3.24 Distribution of the top 10 cancer sites in terms of mortality for females in peri-urban areas of Beijing, 2017

（撰稿 刘硕，校稿 李慧超）

5 各部位恶性肿瘤的发病和死亡
Cancer incidences and mortalities by site

5.1 口腔和咽 (C00-10, C12-14)

2017 年，北京市口腔癌和咽癌新发病例数为 619 例，占全部恶性肿瘤发病的 1.24%，位居恶性肿瘤发病第 19 位；其中男性 388 例，女性 231 例，城区 434 例，郊区 185 例。口腔癌和咽癌发病率为 4.55/10 万，中标发病率为 2.40/10 万，世标发病率为 2.34/10 万；男性世标发病率为女性的 1.78 倍，城区世标发病率为郊区的 1.26 倍。0~74 岁累积发病率为 0.26%（表 5.1.1）。

5.1 Oral cavity & Pharynx (C00-10, C12-14)

There were 619 new cases diagnosed as oral cavity and pharynx cancer (388 males and 231 females, 434 in urban areas and 185 in peri-urban areas), accounting for 1.24% of new cases of all cancers in 2017. Oral cavity and pharynx cancer was the 19th common cancer in Beijing. The crude incidence rate was 4.55 per 100,000, with an ASR China and ASR World of 2.40 and 2.34 per 100,000, respectively. The incidence of ASR World were 78% higher in males than in females and 26% higher in urban areas than in peri-urban areas. The cumulative incidence rate for subjects aged 0 to 74 years was 0.26% (Table 5.1.1).

表 5.1.1 2017 年北京市户籍居民口腔癌和咽癌发病情况
Table 5.1.1 Incidence of oral cavity and pharynx cancer in Beijing, 2017

地区 Areas	性别 Sex	例数 No.cases	粗率 Crude rate (1/10^5)	构成比 Freq.（%）	中标率 ASR China (1/10^5)	世标率 ASR World (1/10^5)	累积率 Cumulative rate (0~74, %)	顺位 Rank
全市 All areas	合计 Both	619	4.55	1.24	2.40	2.34	0.26	19
	男性 Male	388	5.71	1.57	2.99	3.01	0.35	14
	女性 Female	231	3.39	0.91	1.81	1.69	0.19	17
城区 Urban areas	合计 Both	434	5.14	1.32	2.60	2.54	0.29	18
	男性 Male	260	6.18	1.61	3.13	3.17	0.36	14
	女性 Female	174	4.11	1.03	2.04	1.90	0.21	17
郊区 Peri-urban areas	合计 Both	185	3.58	1.08	2.06	2.01	0.23	19
	男性 Male	128	4.96	1.48	2.77	2.76	0.32	15
	女性 Female	57	2.20	0.68	1.39	1.30	0.14	18

2017 年，北京市口腔癌和咽癌死亡病例数为 319 例，占全部恶性肿瘤死亡的 1.22%，位居恶性肿瘤死亡第 18 位；其中男性 225 例，女性 94 例，城区 203 例，郊区 116 例。口腔癌和咽癌死亡率为 2.34/10 万，中标死亡率为 1.04/10 万，世标死亡率为 1.05/10 万；男性世标死亡率为女性的 3.11 倍，郊区世标死亡率为城区的 1.15 倍。0~74 岁累积死亡率为 0.12%（表 5.1.2）。

A total of 319 cases died of oral cavity and pharynx cancer (225 males and 94 females, 203 in urban areas and 116 in peri-urban areas), accounting for 1.22% of all cancer deaths in 2017. Oral cavity and pharynx cancer was the 18th leading cause of cancer deaths in all cancers. The crude mortality rate was 2.34 per 100,000, with an ASR China and an ASR World of 1.04 and 1.05 per 100,000, respectively. The ASR World for mortality was 211% higher in males than in females and 15% higher in peri-urban areas than in urban areas. The cumulative mortality rate for subjects aged 0 to 74 years was 0.12% (Table 5.1.2).

表 5.1.2 2017 年北京市户籍居民口腔癌和咽癌死亡情况
Table 5.1.2 Mortality of oral cavity and pharynx cancer in Beijing, 2017

地区 Areas	性别 Sex	例数 No.deaths	粗率 Crude rate （1/10^5）	构成比 Freq.（%）	中标率 ASR China （1/10^5）	世标率 ASR World （1/10^5）	累积率 Cumulative rate（0~74, %）	顺位 Rank
全市 All areas	合计 Both	319	2.34	1.22	1.04	1.05	0.12	18
	男性 Male	225	3.31	1.45	1.57	1.60	0.19	14
	女性 Female	94	1.38	0.89	0.52	0.51	0.05	17
城区 Urban areas	合计 Both	203	2.41	1.20	0.98	0.99	0.11	18
	男性 Male	140	3.33	1.40	1.44	1.48	0.18	13
	女性 Female	63	1.49	0.90	0.52	0.51	0.05	17
郊区 Peri-urban areas	合计 Both	116	2.24	1.28	1.13	1.14	0.13	18
	男性 Male	85	3.29	1.54	1.75	1.78	0.21	14
	女性 Female	31	1.20	0.87	0.52	0.52	0.06	18

北京市口腔癌和咽癌世标发病率由 2008 年的 2.03/10 万上升到 2017 年的 2.34/10 万，年均变化百分比（annual percentage change, APC）为 1.77%（P=0.005）；男性和女性发病 10 年间年均变化百分比分别为 2.04%（P=0.018）和 1.27%（P=0.137）。北京市口腔癌和咽癌世标

The incidence of ASR World of oral cavity and pharynx cancer increased from 2.03 per 100,000 in 2008 to 2.34 per 100,000 in 2017; the APC of ASR World for incidence was 1.77% (P=0.005). The APC of ASR World for incidence of oral cavity and pharynx cancer in males and females were 2.04% (P=0.018) and 1.27% (P=0.137), respectively. The mortality of ASR World of oral cavity and pharynx cancer increased from 0.92 per 100,000 in 2008 to 1.05 per 100,000 in

死亡率由 2008 年的 0.92/10 万上升到 2017 年的 1.05/10 万,年均变化百分比为 2.18%(*P*<0.001);男性和女性死亡 10 年间年均变化百分比分别为 2.80%(*P*<0.001)和 0.39%(*P*=0.820)。

口腔癌和咽癌年龄别发病率和死亡率在 40 岁以前均较低,40 岁以后快速上升,男性上升速度高于女性(图 5.1.1 至图 5.1.6)。除 75~79 岁年龄组女性发病率略高于男性外,40 岁以上年龄组男性口腔癌和咽癌发病率及死亡率均高于女性,男性和女性发病率均在 75~79 岁组达到高峰,死亡率均在 85 岁及以上年龄组达到高峰(图 5.1.1 和图 5.1.4)。城区和郊区年龄别发病率、死亡率变化有一定差别,但总体趋势相同,郊区波动较为明显(图 5.1.2 和图 5.1.3,图 5.1.5 和图 5.1.6)。

2017; the APC of ASR World for mortality was 2.18% (*P*<0.001). The APC of ASR World for mortality of oral cavity and pharynx cancer in males and females were 2.80% (*P*<0.001) and 0.39% (*P*=0.820), respectively.

The age-specific incidence and mortality rates of oral cavity and pharynx cancer were relatively low in people below 40 years old, and the rates increased sharply in people older than that, and the growth rates were higher in males than females (Figure 5.1.1- 5.1.6). Except the incidence rate was slightly higher in females than that in males at the age group of 75-79 years, the incidence and mortality rates in males were consistently higher than that in females after 40 years old. The age-specific incidence rates for both males and females peaked at the age group of 75-79 years, and the age-specific mortality rates for both sexes peaked at the age group of 85 years and above (Figure 5.1.1, Figure 5.1.4). There were some differences in age-specific incidence and mortality rates between urban and peri-urban areas, but the overall trends were the same. The distributions of age-specific incidence and mortality rates in peri-urban areas showed some fluctuations (Figure 5.1.2-5.1.3, Figure 5.1.5-5.1.6).

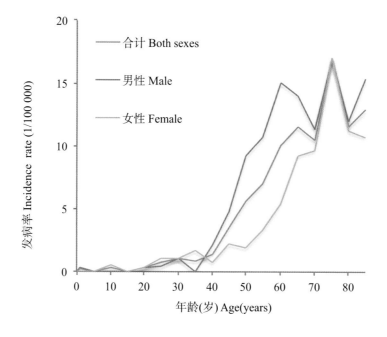

图 5.1.1 2017 年北京市户籍居民口腔癌和咽癌年龄别发病率
Figure 5.1.1 Age-specific incidence rates of oral cavity and pharynx cancer in Beijing, 2017

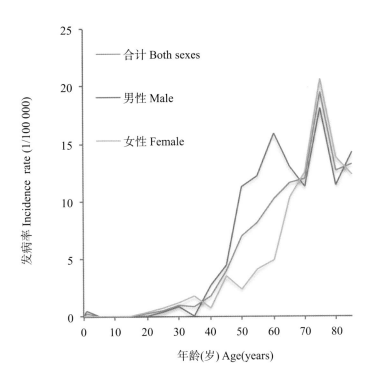

图 5.1.2 2017 年北京市城区户籍居民口腔癌和咽癌年龄别发病率
Figure 5.1.2 Age-specific incidence rates of oral cavity and pharynx cancer in urban areas of Beijing, 2017

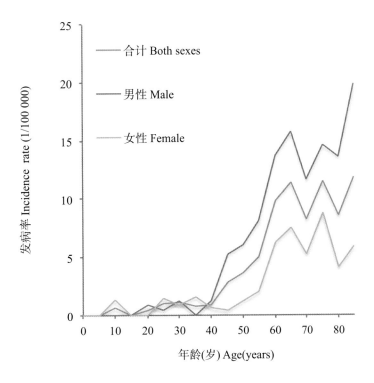

图 5.1.3 2017 年北京市郊区户籍居民口腔癌和咽癌年龄别发病率
Figure 5.1.3 Age-specific incidence rates of oral cavity and pharynx cancer in peri-urban areas of Beijing, 2017

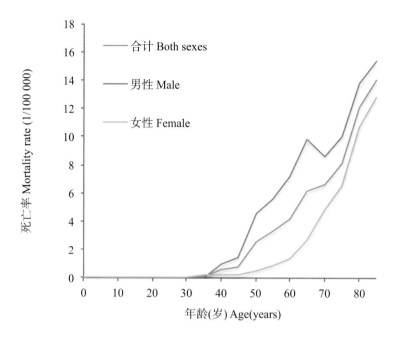

图 5.1.4 2017 年北京市户籍居民口腔癌和咽癌年龄别死亡率
Figure 5.1.4 Age-specific mortality rates of oral cavity and pharynx cancer in Beijing, 2017

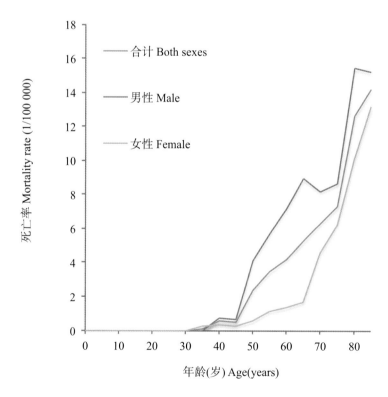

图 5.1.5 2017 年北京市城区户籍居民口腔癌和咽癌年龄别死亡率
Figure 5.1.5 Age-specific mortality rates of oral cavity and pharynx cancer in urban areas of Beijing, 2017

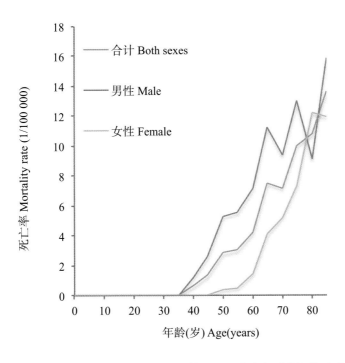

图 5.1.6 2017 年北京市郊区户籍居民口腔癌和咽癌年龄别死亡率

Figure 5.1.6 Age-specific mortality rates of oral cavity and pharynx cancer in peri-urban areas of Beijing, 2017

全部口腔癌和咽癌新发病例中，有明确亚部位的病例数占 95.96%。其中口腔是最常见的发病部位，占 37.32%；其次是舌、唾液腺和下咽，分别占 21.16%、13.25% 和 12.28%（图 5.1.7）。

About 95.96% cases were assigned to specified categories of oral cavity and pharynx cancer site. Among those, mouth cancer was the most common site, accounting for 37.32% of all cases, followed by the tongue (21.16%), the salivary glands (13.25%) and the hypopharynx (12.28%) (Figure 5.1.7).

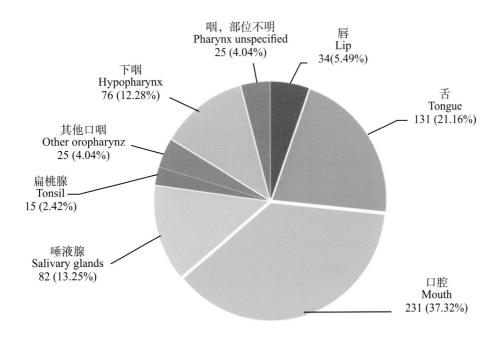

图 5.1.7 2017 年北京市户籍居民口腔癌和咽癌亚部位分布情况

Figure 5.1.7 Subsite distribution of oral cavity and pharynx cancer in Beijing, 2017

（撰稿 刘硕，校稿 张倩）

5.2 鼻咽（C11）[5]

2017 年，北京市鼻咽癌新发病例数为 80 例，占全部恶性肿瘤发病的 0.16%，位居恶性肿瘤发病第 23 位；其中男性 56 例，女性 24 例，城区 48 例，郊区 32 例。鼻咽癌发病率为 0.59/10 万，中标发病率为 0.36/10 万，世标发病率为 0.33/10 万；男性世标发病率为女性的 3.18 倍，郊区世标发病率为城区的 1.09 倍。0~74 岁累积发病率为 0.04%（表 5.2.1）。

5.2 Nasopharynx (C11)

There were 80 new cases diagnosed as nasopharyngeal cancer (56 males and 24 females, 48 in urban areas and 32 in peri-urban areas), accounting for 0.16% of new cases of all cancers in 2017. Nasopharyngeal cancer was the 23rd common cancer in Beijing. The crude incidence rate was 0.59 per 100,000, with an ASR China and an ASR World of 0.36 and 0.33 per 100,000, respectively. The ASR World for incidence was 218% higher in males than in females and 9% higher in peri-urban areas than in urban areas. The cumulative incidence rate for subjects aged 0 to 74 years was 0.04% (Table 5.2.1).

表 5.2.1 2017 年北京市户籍居民鼻咽癌发病情况
Table 5.2.1 Incidence of nasopharyngeal cancer in Beijing, 2017

地区 Areas	性别 Sex	例数 No. cases	粗率 Crude rate (1/10⁵)	构成比 Freq.（%）	中标率 ASR China （1/10⁵）	世标率 ASR World （1/10⁵）	累积率 Cumulative rate(0~74, %)	顺位 Rank
全市 All areas	合计 Both	80	0.59	0.16	0.36	0.33	0.04	23
	男性 Male	56	0.82	0.23	0.56	0.51	0.06	19
	女性 Female	24	0.35	0.09	0.16	0.16	0.02	22
城区 Urban areas	合计 Both	48	0.57	0.15	0.35	0.32	0.03	25
	男性 Male	32	0.76	0.20	0.56	0.49	0.05	19
	女性 Female	16	0.38	0.09	0.15	0.15	0.02	22
郊区 Peri-urban areas	合计 Both	32	0.62	0.19	0.38	0.35	0.04	23
	男性 Male	24	0.93	0.28	0.59	0.54	0.06	19
	女性 Female	8	0.31	0.09	0.18	0.17	0.02	22

2017 年，北京市鼻咽癌死亡病例数为 86 例，占全部恶性肿瘤死亡的 0.33%，位居恶性肿瘤死亡第 23 位；其中男性 68 例，女性 18 例，城区 63 例，

A total of 86 cases died of nasopharyngeal cancer (68 males and 18 females, 63 in urban areas and 23 in peri-urban areas), accounting for 0.33% of all cancer deaths in 2017. Nasopharyngeal cancer was the 23rd leading

---

5. 因北京市鼻咽癌发病和死亡例数较少，因此本节不包含年龄别发病率和死亡率的统计数据和图表。
  Because of few nasopharyngeal cance cases and deaths occured in Beijing in 2017, this section does not contain statistical data and charts on age-specific incidence and mortality rates.

郊区 23 例。鼻咽癌死亡率为 0.63/10 万，中标死亡率为 0.38/10 万，世标死亡率为 0.36/10 万；男性世标死亡率为女性的 5.48 倍，城区世标死亡率为郊区的 1.07 倍。0~74 岁累积死亡率为 0.04%（表5.2.2）。

cause of cancer deaths in all cancers. The crude mortality rate was 0.63 per 100,000, with an ASR China and an ASR World of 0.38 and 0.36 per 100,000, respectively. The ASR World for mortality was 448% higher in males than in females and 7% higher in urban areas than in peri-urban areas. The cumulative mortality rate for subjects aged 0 to 74 years was 0.04% (Table 5.2.2).

表 5.2.2 2017 年北京市户籍居民鼻咽癌死亡情况
Table 5.2.2 Mortality of nasopharyngeal cancer in Beijing, 2017

地区 Areas	性别 Sex	例数 No. deaths	粗率 Crude rate （1/10⁵）	构成比 Freq.（%）	中标率 ASR China （1/10⁵）	世标率 ASR World （1/10⁵）	累积率 Cumulative rate（0~74，%）	顺位 Rank
全市 All areas	合计 Both	86	0.63	0.33	0.38	0.36	0.04	23
	男性 Male	68	1.00	0.44	0.65	0.62	0.06	17
	女性 Female	18	0.26	0.17	0.11	0.11	0.01	22
城区 Urban areas	合计 Both	63	0.75	0.37	0.39	0.37	0.04	22
	男性 Male	49	1.16	0.49	0.66	0.62	0.07	16
	女性 Female	14	0.33	0.20	0.12	0.12	0.01	22
郊区 Peri-urban areas	合计 Both	23	0.44	0.25	0.35	0.34	0.03	23
	男性 Male	19	0.74	0.34	0.61	0.60	0.06	18
	女性 Female	4	0.15	0.11	0.10	0.09	0.01	22

北京市鼻咽癌世标发病率由 2008 年的 0.53/10 万下降到 2017 年的 0.33/10 万，年均变化百分比为 −5.19%（P=0.011）；男性和女性发病 10 年间年均变化百分比分别为 −4.77%（P=0.015）和 −6.41%（P=0.026）。北京市鼻咽癌世标死亡率由 2008 年的 0.41/10 万下降到 2017 年的 0.36/10 万，年均变化百分比为 −1.23%（P=0.250）；男性和女性死亡 10 年间年均变化百分比分别为 −0.66%（P=0.655）和 −2.98%（P=0.423）。

The ASR World for incidence of nasopharyngeal cancer decreased from 0.53 per 100,000 in 2008 to 0.33 per 100,000 in 2017; the APC of ASR World for incidence was −5.19% (P=0.011). The APCs of ASR World for incidence of nasopharyngeal cancer in males and females were −4.77% (P=0.015) and −6.41% (P=0.026), respectively. The ASR World for mortality of nasopharyngeal cancer decreased from 0.41 per 100,000 in 2008 to 0.36 per 100,000 in 2017; the APC of ASR World for mortality was −1.23% (P=0.250). The APCs of ASR World for mortality of nasopharyngeal cancer in males and females were −0.66% (P=0.655) and −2.98% (P=0.423), respectively.

（撰稿 程杨杨，校稿 张希）

5.3 食管 (C15)

2017 年，北京市食管癌新发病例数为 1 183 例，占全部恶性肿瘤发病的 2.36%，位居恶性肿瘤发病第 16 位；其中男性 964 例，女性 219 例，城区 659 例，郊区 524 例。食管癌发病率为 8.69/10 万，中标发病率为 3.71/10 万，世标发病率为 3.78/10 万；男性世标发病率为女性的 5.99 倍，郊区世标发病率为城区的 1.51 倍。0~74 岁累积发病率为 0.44%（表 5.3.1）。

5.3 Esophagus (C15)

There were 1,183 new cases diagnosed as esophageal cancer (964 males and 219 females, 659 in urban areas and 524 in peri-urban areas), accounting for 2.36% of new cases of all cancers in 2017. Esophageal cancer was the 16th common cancer in Beijing. The crude incidence rate was 8.69 per 100,000, with an ASR China and an ASR World of 3.71 and 3.78 per 100,000, respectively. The ASR World for incidence was 499% higher in males than in females and 51% higher in peri-urban areas than in urban areas. The cumulative incidence rate for subjects aged 0 to 74 years was 0.44% (Table 5.3.1).

表 5.3.1 2017 年北京市户籍居民食管癌发病情况
Table 5.3.1 Incidence of esophageal cancer in Beijing, 2017

地区 Areas	性别 Sex	例数 No. cases	粗率 Crude rate （1/10⁵）	构成比 Freq.（%）	中标率 ASR China （1/10⁵）	世标率 ASR World （1/10⁵）	累积率 Cumulative rate(0~74, %）	顺位 Rank
全市 All areas	合计 Both	1 183	8.69	2.36	3.71	3.78	0.44	16
	男性 Male	964	14.19	3.89	6.47	6.61	0.80	9
	女性 Female	219	3.21	0.86	1.11	1.10	0.10	18
城区 Urban areas	合计 Both	659	7.81	2.00	3.15	3.22	0.37	16
	男性 Male	519	12.33	3.22	5.34	5.50	0.66	11
	女性 Female	140	3.31	0.83	1.05	1.03	0.09	18
郊区 Peri-urban areas	合计 Both	524	10.14	3.07	4.81	4.88	0.55	12
	男性 Male	445	17.24	5.15	8.64	8.77	1.02	5
	女性 Female	79	3.05	0.94	1.25	1.26	0.12	17

2017 年，北京市食管癌死亡病例数为 1 058 例，占全部恶性肿瘤死亡的 4.06%，位居恶性肿瘤死亡第 8 位；其中男性 856 例，女性 202 例，城区

A total of 1,058 cases died of esophageal cancer (856 males and 202 females, 590 in urban areas and 468 in peri-urban areas), accounting for 4.06% of all cancer deaths in 2017. Esophageal cancer was the

590 例，郊区 468 例。食管癌死亡率为 7.77/10 万，中标死亡率为 3.11/10 万，世标死亡率为 3.16/10 万；男性世标死亡率为女性的 6.21 倍，郊区世标死亡率为城区的 1.60 倍。0~74 岁累积死亡率为 0.35%（表 5.3.2）。

8th leading cause of cancer deaths in all cancers. The crude mortality rate was 7.77 per 100,000, with an ASR China and an ASR World of 3.11 and 3.16 per 100,000, respectively. The ASR World for mortality was 521% higher in males than in females and 60% higher in peri-urban areas than in urban areas. The cumulative mortality rate for subjects aged 0 to 74 years was 0.35% (Table 5.3.2).

表 5.3.2　2017 年北京市户籍居民食管癌死亡情况
Table 5.3.2 Mortality of esophageal cancer in Beijing, 2017

地区 Areas	性别 Sex	例数 No. deaths	粗率 Crude rate (1/10⁵)	构成比 Freq.（%）	中标率 ASR China (1/10⁵)	世标率 ASR World (1/10⁵)	累积率 Cumulative rate(0~74, %)	顺位 Rank
全市 All areas	合计 Both	1 058	7.77	4.06	3.11	3.16	0.35	8
	男性 Male	856	12.60	5.52	5.48	5.57	0.65	5
	女性 Female	202	2.96	1.92	0.91	0.90	0.07	15
城区 Urban areas	合计 Both	590	6.99	3.47	2.58	2.64	0.29	10
	男性 Male	462	10.97	4.63	4.45	4.58	0.54	6
	女性 Female	128	3.03	1.83	0.80	0.79	0.05	16
郊区 Peri-urban areas	合计 Both	468	9.05	5.16	4.20	4.22	0.45	6
	男性 Male	394	15.26	7.14	7.55	7.61	0.84	5
	女性 Female	74	2.86	2.09	1.13	1.13	0.09	14

北京市食管癌世标发病率由 2008 年的 5.53/10 万下降到 2017 年的 3.78/10 万，年均变化百分比为 -4.64%（P<0.001）；男性和女性发病 10 年间年均变化百分比分别为 -4.04%（P<0.001）和 -7.69%（P<0.001）。北京市食管癌世标死亡率由 2008 年的 4.32/10 万下降到 2017 年的 3.16/10 万，年均变化百分比为 -4.10%

The incidence of ASR World of esophageal cancer decreased from 5.53 per 100,000 in 2008 to 3.78 per 100,000 in 2017; the APC of ASR World for incidence of was -4.64% (P<0.001). The APCs of ASR World for incidence of esophageal cancer in males and females were -4.04% (P<0.001) and -7.69% (P<0.001), respectively. The mortality of ASR World of esophageal cancer decreased from 4.32 per 100,000 in 2008 to 3.16 per 100,000 in 2017; the APC of ASR World for mortality of was -4.10% (P<0.001). The APCs of ASR

（*P*<0.001）；男性和女性死亡 10 年间年均变化百分比分别为 -3.53%（*P*<0.001）和 -6.95%（*P*<0.001）。

食管癌年龄别发病率和死亡率在 40 岁以前均较低，40 岁以后快速上升，男性上升速度高于女性（图 5.3.1 至图 5.3.6）。40 岁以上年龄组男性食管癌发病率和死亡率均高于女性，男性和女性发病率与死亡率均在 85 岁及以上年龄组达到高峰（图 5.3.1 和图 5.3.4）。城区和郊区年龄别发病率、死亡率变化有一定差别，但总体趋势相同，城区波动较为明显（图 5.3.2 和图 5.3.3，图 5.3.5 和图 5.3.6）。

World for mortality of esophageal cancer in males and females were -3.53% (*P*<0.001) and -6.95% (*P*<0.001), respectively.

The age-specific incidence and mortality rates of esophageal cancer were relatively low in people below 40 years old, but the rates increased sharply in people older than that, furthermore the growth rates were higher in males than those in females (Figure 5.3.1-5.3.6). The incidence and mortality rates in males were consistently higher than those in females after 40 years old, and the age-specific incidence and mortality rates for both sexes peaked at the age group of 85 years and above (Figure 5.3.1, Figure 5.3.4). There were some differences in age-specific incidence and mortality rates between urban and peri-urban areas, but the overall trends were same. The age-specific incidence and mortality rates in urban areas showed significant fluctuations (Figure 5.3.2-5.3.3, Figure 5.3.5-5.3.6).

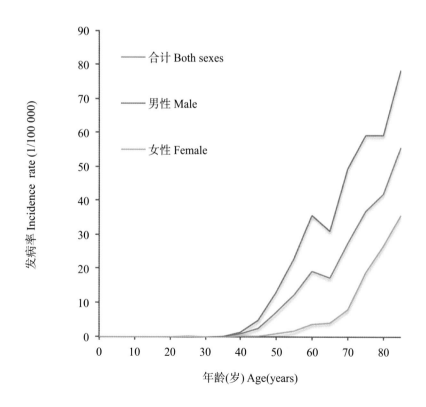

图 5.3.1 2017 年北京市户籍居民食管癌年龄别发病率
Figure 5.3.1 Age-specific incidence rates of esophageal cancer in Beijing, 2017

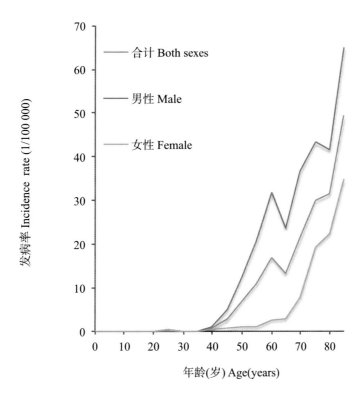

图 5.3.2 2017 年北京市城区户籍居民食管癌年龄别发病率
Figure 5.3.2 Age-specific incidence rates of esophageal cancer in urban areas of Beijing, 2017

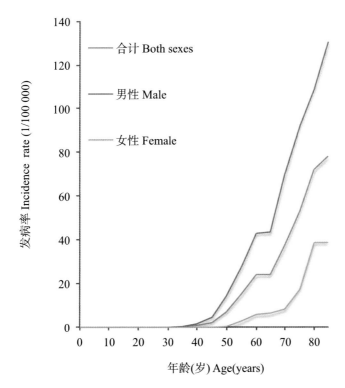

图 5.3.3 2017 年北京市郊区户籍居民食管癌年龄别发病率
Figure 5.3.3 Age-specific incidence rates of esophageal cancer in peri-urban areas of Beijing, 2017

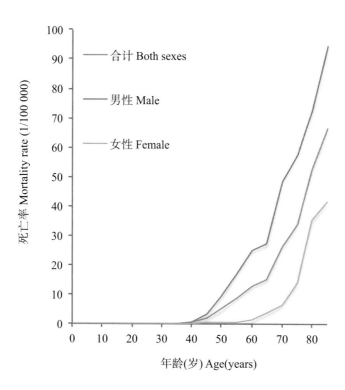

图 5.3.4 2017 年北京市户籍居民食管癌年龄别死亡率

Figure 5.3.4 Age-specific mortality rates of esophageal cancer in Beijing, 2017

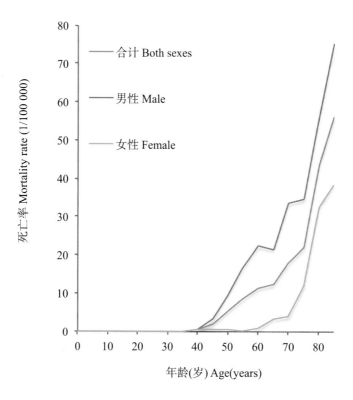

图 5.3.5 2017 年北京市城区户籍居民食管癌年龄别死亡率

Figure 5.3.5 Age-specific mortality rates of esophageal cancer in urban areas of Beijing, 2017

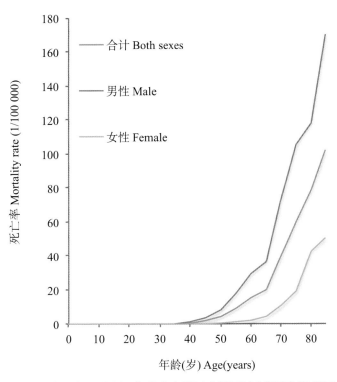

图 5.3.6　2017 年北京市郊区户籍居民食管癌年龄别死亡率

Figure 5.3.6 Age-specific mortality rates of esophageal cancer in peri-urban areas of Beijing, 2017

2017 年，北京市食管癌世标发病率和死亡率在 16 个辖区间存在显著差异，郊区发病率和死亡率均高于城区（图 5.3.7 和图 5.3.8）。

In 2017, there were significant differences between the 16 districts in ASR World for incidence and mortality of esophageal cancer in Beijing. The incidence and mortality rates were higher in peri-urban areas than in urban areas (Figure 5.3.7-5.3.8).

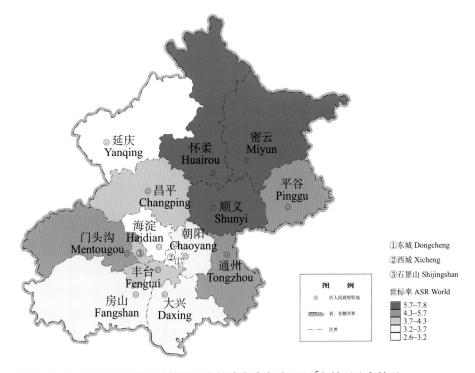

图 5.3.7　2017 年北京市户籍居民食管癌发病率（1/10⁵）地区分布情况

Figure 5.3.7 Incidence rates of esophageal cancer by district in Beijing, 2017 (1/10⁵)

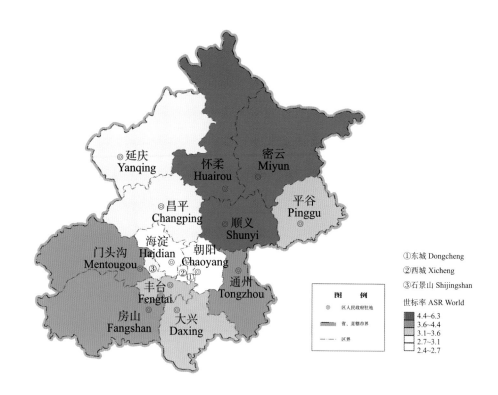

图 5.3.8 2017 年北京市户籍居民食管癌死亡率（1/10⁵）地区分布情况
Figure 5.3.8 Mortality rates of esophageal cancer by district in Beijing, 2017 (1/10⁵)

全部食管癌新发病例中，有明确亚部位病例数占 34.83%。其中食管中段是最常见的发病部位，占 87.62%；其后依次为食管下段、交搭跨越、食管上段，分别占 8.01%、2.43% 和 1.94%（图5.3.9）。

About 34.83% cases were assigned to specified categories of esophageal cancer site. Among those, the middle third of the esophagus was the most common site, accounting for 87.62% of all cases, followed by the lower third (8.01%), the overlapping (2.43%) and the upper third esophagus (1.94%) (Figure 5.3.9).

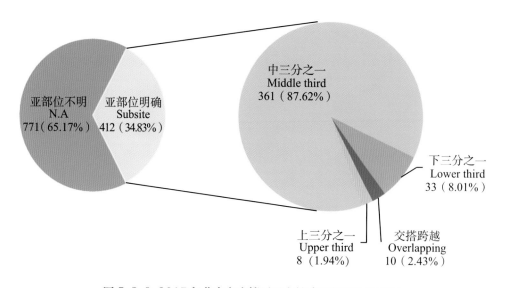

图 5.3.9 2017 年北京市户籍居民食管癌亚部位分布情况
Figure 5.3.9 Subsite distribution of esophageal cancer in Beijing, 2017

（撰稿 张倩，校稿 李晴雨）

5.4 胃（C16）

2017 年，北京市胃癌新发病例数为 2 471 例，占全部恶性肿瘤发病的 4.94%，位居恶性肿瘤发病第 7 位；其中男性 1 667 例，女性 804 例，城区 1 701 例，郊区 770 例。胃癌发病率为 18.16/10 万，中标发病率为 8.52/10 万，世标发病率为 8.33/10 万；男性世标发病率为女性的 2.15 倍，城区世标发病率为郊区的 1.13 倍。0~74 岁累积发病率为 0.96%（表 5.4.1）。

5.4 Stomach (C16)

There were 2,471 new cases diagnosed as stomach cancer (1,667 males and 804 females, 1,701 in urban areas and 770 in peri-urban areas), accounting for 4.94% of new cases of all cancers in 2017. Stomach cancer was the 7th common cancer in Beijing. The crude incidence rate was 18.16 per 100,000, with an ASR China and an ASR World of 8.52 and 8.33 per 100,000, respectively. The ASR World for incidence was 115% higher in males than in females and 13% higher in urban areas than in peri-urban areas. The cumulative incidence rate for subjects aged 0 to 74 years was 0.96% (Table 5.4.1).

表 5.4.1 2017 年北京市户籍居民胃癌发病情况
Table 5.4.1 Incidence of stomach cancer in Beijing, 2017

地区 Areas	性别 Sex	例数 No. cases	粗率 Crude rate (1/10^5)	构成比 Freq.（%）	中标率 ASR China (1/10^5)	世标率 ASR World (1/10^5)	累积率 Cumulative rate(0~74, %)	顺位 Rank
全市 All areas	合计 Both	2 471	18.16	4.94	8.52	8.33	0.96	7
	男性 Male	1 667	24.55	6.73	11.65	11.52	1.37	4
	女性 Female	804	11.79	3.18	5.62	5.37	0.58	8
城区 Urban areas	合计 Both	1 701	20.15	5.16	8.90	8.72	1.02	7
	男性 Male	1 122	26.65	6.96	11.86	11.72	1.41	4
	女性 Female	579	13.69	3.43	6.18	5.93	0.66	6
郊区 Peri-urban areas	合计 Both	770	14.89	4.51	7.86	7.68	0.87	8
	男性 Male	545	21.11	6.31	11.26	11.18	1.32	4
	女性 Female	225	8.69	2.67	4.70	4.45	0.45	10

2017 年，北京市胃癌死亡病例数为 1 715 例，占全部恶性肿瘤死亡的 6.58%，位居恶性肿瘤死亡第 5 位；其中男性 1 163 例，女性 552 例，城区1 155 例，郊区 560 例。胃癌死亡率为 12.60/10 万，中标死亡率为 5.33/10 万，世标死亡率为 5.18/10万；男性世标死亡率为女性的 2.09 倍，郊区世标死亡率为城区的 1.02 倍。0~74 岁累积死亡率为0.53%（表 5.4.2）。

A total of 1,715 cases died of stomach cancer (1,163 males and 552 females, 1,155 in urban areas and 560 in peri-urban areas), accounting for 6.58% of all cancer deaths in 2017. Stomach cancer was the 5th leading cause of cancer deaths in all cancers. The crude mortality rate was 12.60 per 100,000, with an ASR China and an ASR World of 5.33 and 5.18 per 100,000, respectively. The ASR World for mortality was 109% higher in males than in females and 2% higher in peri-urban areas than in urban areas. The cumulative mortality rate for subjects aged 0 to 74 years was 0.53% (Table 5.4.2).

表 5.4.2 2017 年北京市户籍居民胃癌死亡情况
Table 5.4.2 Mortality of stomach cancer in Beijing, 2017

地区 Areas	性别 Sex	例数 No. deaths	粗率 Crude rate （1/10^5）	构成比 Freq.（%）	中标率 ASR China （1/10^5）	世标率 ASR World （1/10^5）	累积率 Cumulative rate(0~74,%)	顺位 Rank
全市 All areas	合计 Both	1 715	12.60	6.58	5.33	5.18	0.53	5
	男性 Male	1 163	17.12	7.50	7.29	7.14	0.75	4
	女性 Female	552	8.10	5.23	3.57	3.41	0.33	6
城区 Urban areas	合计 Both	1 155	13.68	6.80	5.26	5.14	0.53	5
	男性 Male	768	18.24	7.69	7.04	6.91	0.73	4
	女性 Female	387	9.15	5.53	3.68	3.56	0.35	6
郊区 Peri-urban areas	合计 Both	560	10.83	6.18	5.45	5.24	0.52	5
	男性 Male	395	15.30	7.16	7.74	7.57	0.76	4
	女性 Female	165	6.38	4.66	3.37	3.14	0.29	5

北京市胃癌世标发病率由 2008 年的 9.83/10 万下降到 2017 年的 8.33/10 万，10 年间发病率平均变化百分比为 -2.14%，发病率呈下降趋势（P<0.001）；男性和女性 10 年间发病率年均变

The ASR World for incidence of stomach cancer decreased from 9.83 per 100,000 in 2008 to 8.33 per 100,000 in 2017; the APC of ASR World for incidence was -2.14% (P<0.001). The APCs of ASR World for incidence of stomach cancer in males and females were -2.19% (P<0.001) and -2.13% (P=0.002),

化百分比分别为 -2.19%（P<0.001）和 -2.13%（P=0.002）。北京市胃癌世标死亡率由 2008 年的 6.94/10 万下降到 2017 年的 5.18/10 万，年均变化百分比为 -3.30%（P<0.001）；男性和女性 10 年间死亡率年均变化百分比分别为 -3.60%（P<0.001）和 -2.66%（P<0.001）。

　　胃癌年龄别发病率和死亡率在 40 岁以前均较低，40 岁以后快速上升，男性上升速度高于女性（图 5.4.1 至图 5.4.6）。男性和女性发病率均在 80~84 岁年龄组达到高峰，男性死亡率在 80~84 岁年龄组达到高峰，女性死亡率在 85 岁及以上年龄组达到高峰（图 5.4.1 和图 5.4.4）。城区和郊区年龄别发病率、死亡率变化有一定差别，但总体趋势相同（图 5.4.2 和图 5.4.3，图 5.4.5 和图 5.4.6）。

respectively. The ASR World for mortality of stomach cancer decreased from 6.94 per 100,000 in 2008 to 5.18 per 100,000 in 2017; the APC of ASR World for mortality was -3.30% (P <0.001). The APCs of ASR World for mortality of stomach cancer in males and females were -3.60% (P<0.001) and -2.66% (P<0.001), respectively.

The age-specific incidence and mortality rates of stomach cancer were relatively low in people below 40 years old, and the rates increased sharply in people older than that; furthermore, the growth rates were higher in males than females (Figure 5.4.1-5.4.6). The age-specific incidence rates for both males and females peaked at the age group of 80-84 years, and the age-specific mortality rates peaked in the age group of 75-79 years in males and the age group of 85 years and above in females (Figure 5.4.1, Figure 5.4.4). There were some differences in age-specific incidence and mortality rates between urban and peri-urban areas, but the overall trends were the same (Figure 5.4.2-5.4.3, Figure 5.4.5-5.4.6).

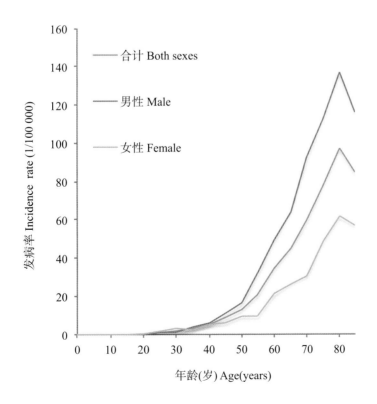

图 5.4.1 2017 年北京市户籍居民胃癌年龄别发病率
Figure 5.4.1 Age-specific incidence rates of stomach cancer in Beijing, 2017

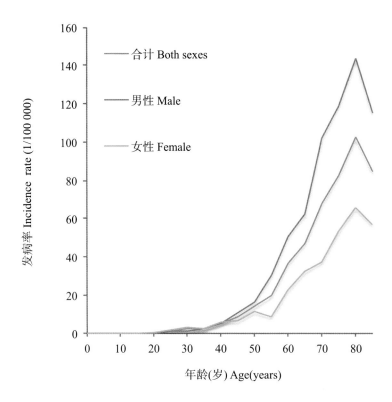

图 5.4.2 2017 年北京市城区户籍居民胃癌年龄别发病率
Figure 5.4.2 Age-specific incidence rates of stomach cancer in urban areas of Beijing, 2017

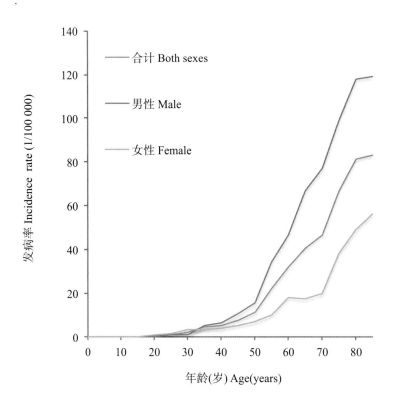

图 5.4.3 2017 年北京市郊区户籍居民胃癌年龄别发病率
Figure 5.4.3 Age-specific incidence rates of stomach cancer in peri-urban areas of Beijing, 2017

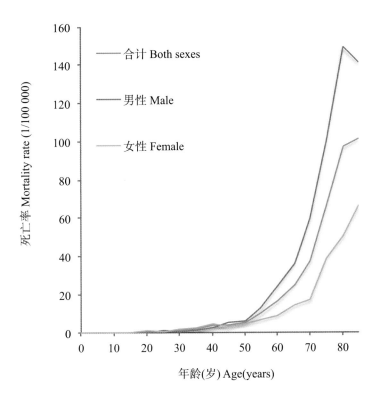

图 5.4.4 2017 年北京市户籍居民胃癌年龄别死亡率
Figure 5.4.4 Age-specific mortality rates of stomach cancer in Beijing, 2017

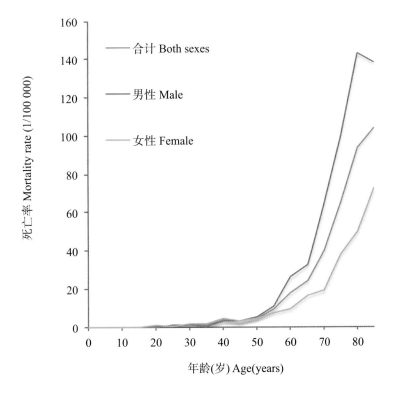

图 5.4.5 2017 年北京市城区户籍居民胃癌年龄别死亡率
Figure 5.4.5 Age-specific mortality rates of stomach cancer in urban areas of Beijing, 2017

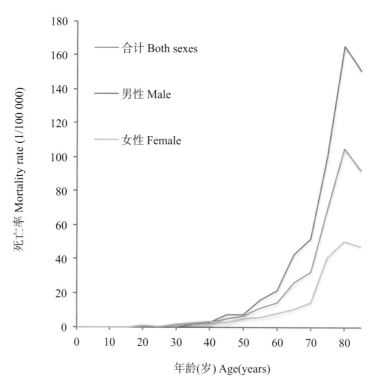

图 5.4.6　2017 年北京市郊区户籍居民胃癌年龄别死亡率
Figure 5.4.6 Age-specific mortality rates of stomach cancer in peri-urban areas of Beijing, 2017

2017 年，北京市胃癌世标发病率和死亡率在 16 个辖区间有显著差异，城区发病率高于郊区，郊区死亡率高于城区（图 5.4.7 和图 5.4.8）。

In 2017, there were significant differences between the 16 districts in ASR World for incidence and mortality of stomach cancer in Beijing. The incidence rate was higher in urban areas than in peri-urban areas, while the mortality rate was higher in the peri-urban areas than in urban areas (Figure 5.4.7-5.4.8).

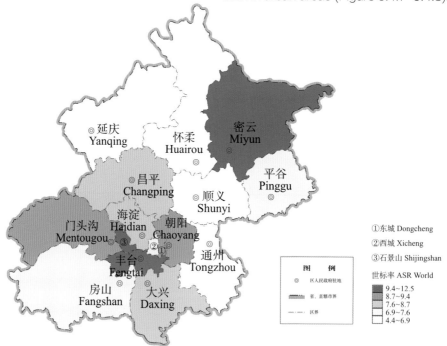

图 5.4.7　2017 年北京市户籍居民胃癌发病率（1/10⁵）地区分布情况
Figure 5.4.7 Incidence rates of stomach cancer by district in Beijing, 2017 (1/10^5)

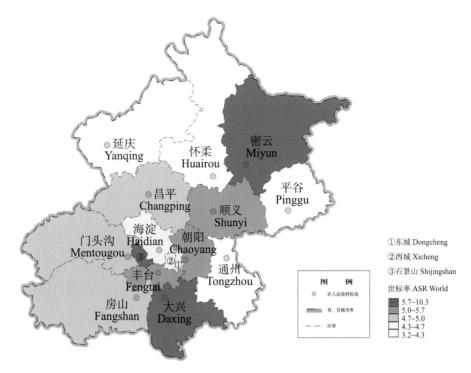

图 5.4.8 2017 年北京市户籍居民胃癌死亡率（$1/10^5$）地区分布情况
Figure 5.4.8 Mortality rates of stomach cancer by district in Beijing, 2017 ($1/10^5$)

全部胃癌新发病例中，有明确亚部位的病例数占 46.46%。其中幽门窦是最常见的胃癌发病亚部位，占 35.89%；其后依次为贲门（29.97%）、胃体（15.16%）、交搭跨越（6.70%）、胃小弯（5.23%）、胃底（4.53%）、幽门（1.74%）和胃大弯（0.78%）（图 5.4.9）。

About 46.46% cases were assigned to specified categories of stomach cancer site. Among those, pyloric antrum was the most common subsite, accounting for 35.89% of all cases, followed by the cardia (29.97%), the body (15.16%), the overlapping (6.70%), the lesser curvature (5.23%), the fundus (4.53%), the pylorus (1.74%), and the greater curvature (0.78%) (Figure 5.4.9).

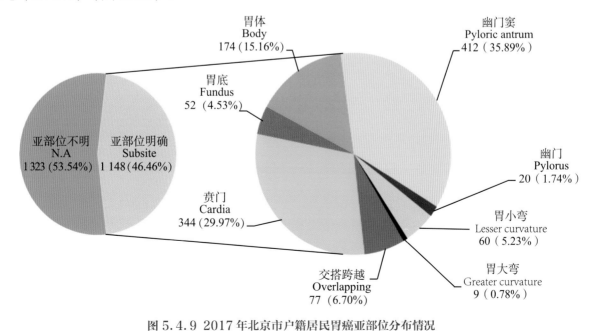

图 5.4.9 2017 年北京市户籍居民胃癌亚部位分布情况
Figure 5.4.9 Subsite distribution of stomach cancer in Beijing, 2017

（撰稿 杨雷，校稿 程杨杨）

5.5 结直肠 (C18-21)

　　2017 年，北京市结直肠癌新发病例数为 6 254 例，占全部恶性肿瘤发病的 12.49%，位居恶性肿瘤发病第 3 位；其中男性 3 620 例，女性 2 634 例，城区 4 337 例，郊区 1 917 例。结直肠癌发病率为 45.95/10 万，中标发病率为 21.38/10 万，世标发病率为 21.10/10 万；男性世标发病率为女性的 1.51 倍，城区世标发病率为郊区的 1.19 倍。0~74 岁累积发病率为 2.51%（表 5.5.1）。

5.5 Colon-rectum (C18-21)

　　There were 6,254 new cases diagnosed as colorectal cancer (3,620 males and 2,634 females, 4,337 in urban areas and 1,917 in peri-urban areas), accounting for 12.49% of new cases of all cancers in 2017. Colorectal cancer was the 3rd common cancer in Beijing. The crude incidence rate was 45.95 per 100,000, with an ASR China and an ASR World of 21.38 and 21.10 per 100,000, respectively. The incidence of ASR World was 51% higher in males than in females and 19% higher in urban areas than in peri-urban areas. The cumulative incidence rate for subjects aged 0 to 74 years was 2.51% (Table 5.5.1).

表 5.5.1　2017 年北京市户籍居民结直肠癌发病情况
Table5.5.1 Incidence of colorectal cancer in Beijing, 2017

地区 Areas	性别 Sex	例数 No. cases	粗率 Crude rate (1/10^5)	构成比 Freq.（%）	中标率 ASR China (1/10^5)	世标率 ASR World (1/10^5)	累积率 Cumulative rate(0~74, %）	顺位 Rank
全市 All areas	合计 Both	6 254	45.95	12.49	21.38	21.10	2.51	3
	男性 Male	3 620	53.30	14.63	25.74	25.55	3.10	2
	女性 Female	2 634	38.63	10.40	17.28	16.91	1.96	4
城区 Urban areas	合计 Both	4 337	51.38	13.14	22.68	22.38	2.68	3
	男性 Male	2 519	59.84	15.63	27.47	27.27	3.34	2
	女性 Female	1 818	42.97	10.77	18.16	17.75	2.06	4
郊区 Peri-urban areas	合计 Both	1 917	37.08	11.23	19.05	18.84	2.24	3
	男性 Male	1 101	42.64	12.74	22.66	22.52	2.70	2
	女性 Female	816	31.53	9.68	15.66	15.40	1.81	4

2017 年，北京市结直肠癌死亡病例数为 2 982 例，占全部恶性肿瘤死亡的 11.45%，位居恶性肿瘤死亡第 2 位；其中男性 1 692 例，女性 1 290 例，城区 2 111 例，郊区 871 例。结直肠癌死亡率为 21.91/10 万，中标死亡率为 8.49/10 万，世标死亡率为 8.40/10 万；男性世标死亡率为女性的 1.51 倍，城区世标死亡率为郊区的 1.11 倍。0~74 岁累积死亡率为 0.82%（表 5.5.2）。

A total of 2,982 cases died of colorectal cancer (1,692 males and 1,290 females, 2,111 in urban areas and 871 in peri-urban areas), accounting for 11.45% of all cancer deaths in 2017. Colorectal cancer was the 2nd leading cause of cancer deaths in all cancers. The crude mortality rate was 21.91 per 100,000, with an ASR China and ASR World of 8.49 and 8.40 per 100,000, respectively. The mortality of ASR World was 51% higher in males than in females and 11% higher in urban areas than in peri-urban areas. The cumulative mortality rate for subjects aged 0 to 74 years was 0.82% (Table 5.5.2).

表 5.5.2 2017 年北京市户籍居民结直肠癌死亡情况
Table 5.5.2 Mortality of colorectal cancer in Beijing, 2017

地区 Areas	性别 Sex	例数 No. deaths	粗率 Crude rate （1/10^5）	构成比 Freq.（%）	中标率 ASR China （1/10^5）	世标率 ASR World （1/10^5）	累积率 Cumulative rate(0~74, %）	顺位 Rank
全市 All areas	合计 Both	2 982	21.91	11.45	8.49	8.40	0.82	2
	男性 Male	1 692	24.91	10.92	10.28	10.19	1.04	2
	女性 Female	1 290	18.92	12.23	6.83	6.74	0.61	2
城区 Urban areas	合计 Both	2 111	25.01	12.43	8.76	8.70	0.85	2
	男性 Male	1 219	28.96	12.21	10.89	10.77	1.08	2
	女性 Female	892	21.08	12.74	6.79	6.76	0.63	2
郊区 Peri-urban areas	合计 Both	871	16.85	9.61	7.98	7.85	0.77	3
	男性 Male	473	18.32	8.57	9.14	9.10	0.96	3
	女性 Female	398	15.38	11.23	6.94	6.71	0.59	2

结肠癌（C18）新发病例数为 3 588 例，占全部恶性肿瘤发病的 7.17%，发病率为 26.36/10 万，中标发病率为 12.14/10 万，世标发病率为 11.85/10 万；其中男性 1 991 例，女性 1 597 例，城区 2 616 例，郊区 972 例。男性世标发病率为女性的 1.39 倍，城区世标发病率为郊区的 1.39 倍。0~74 岁累积发病率为 1.39%（表 5.5.3）。

There were 3,588 new cases diagnosed as colon cancer (C18; 1,991 males and 1,597 females, 2,616 in urban areas and 972 in peri-urban areas), accounting for 7.17% of new cases of all cancers in 2017. The crude incidence rate was 11.85 per 100,000, with an ASR China and an ASR World of 12.14 and 11.85 per 100,000, respectively. The incidence of ASR World was 39% higher in males than in females and 39% higher in urban areas than in peri-urban areas. The cumulative incidence rate for subjects aged 0 to 74 years was 1.39% (Table 5.5.3).

表 5.5.3 2017 年北京市户籍居民结肠癌（C18）发病情况
Table 5.5.3 Incidence of colon cancer(C18) in Beijing, 2017

地区 Areas	性别 Sex	例数 No. cases	粗率 Crude rate （1/10⁵）	构成比 Freq.（%）	中标率 ASR China （1/10⁵）	世标率 ASR World （1/10⁵）	累积率 Cumulative rate(0~74, %)
全市 All areas	合计 Both	3 588	26.36	7.17	12.14	11.85	1.39
	男性 Male	1 991	29.32	8.04	14.17	13.87	1.65
	女性 Female	1 597	23.42	6.31	10.22	9.95	1.14
城区 Urban areas	合计 Both	2 616	30.99	7.93	13.48	13.16	1.56
	男性 Male	1 452	34.49	9.01	15.83	15.49	1.87
	女性 Female	1 164	27.51	6.89	11.27	10.94	1.26
郊区 Peri-urban areas	合计 Both	972	18.80	5.69	9.69	9.49	1.11
	男性 Male	539	20.88	6.24	11.20	10.94	1.28
	女性 Female	433	16.73	5.13	8.26	8.12	0.95

结肠癌（C18）死亡病例数为 1 716 例，占全部恶性肿瘤死亡的 6.59%，死亡率为 12.61/10 万，中标死亡率为 4.83/10 万，世标死亡率为 4.77/10 万；其中男性 912 例，女性 804 例，城区 1 269 例，郊区 447 例。男性世标死亡率为女性的 1.29 倍，城区世标死亡率为郊区的 1.28 倍。0~74 岁累积死亡率为 0.46%（表 5.5.4）。

A total of 1,716 cases died of colon cancer (C18; 912 males and 804 females, 1,269 in urban areas and 447 in peri-urban areas), accounting for 6.59% of all cancer deaths in 2017. The crude mortality rate was 12.61 per 100,000, with an ASR China and an ASR World of 4.83 and 4.77 per 100,000, respectively. The mortality of ASR World was 29% higher in males than in females and 28% higher in urban areas than in peri-urban areas. The cumulative mortality rate for subjects aged 0 to 74 years was 0.46% (Table 5.5.4).

表 5.5.4 2017 年北京市户籍居民结肠癌（C18）死亡情况
Table 5.5.4 Mortality of colon cancer (C18) in Beijing, 2017

地区 Areas	性别 Sex	例数 No. deaths	粗率 Crude rate $(1/10^5)$	构成比 Freq.（%）	中标率 ASR China $(1/10^5)$	世标率 ASR World $(1/10^5)$	累积率 Cumulative rate(0~74, %)
全市 All areas	合计 Both	1 716	12.61	6.59	4.83	4.77	0.46
	男性 Male	912	13.43	5.88	5.44	5.39	0.54
	女性 Female	804	11.79	7.62	4.26	4.19	0.38
城区 Urban areas	合计 Both	1 269	15.04	7.47	5.21	5.16	0.49
	男性 Male	679	16.13	6.80	6.00	5.91	0.58
	女性 Female	590	13.95	8.42	4.47	4.45	0.41
郊区 Peri-urban areas	合计 Both	447	8.65	4.93	4.11	4.02	0.39
	男性 Male	233	9.02	4.22	4.43	4.45	0.46
	女性 Female	214	8.27	6.04	3.83	3.66	0.33

直肠癌（C19-20）新发病例数为 2 643 例，占全部恶性肿瘤发病的 5.28%，发病率为 19.42/10 万，中标发病率为 9.16/10 万，世标发病率为 9.17/10 万；其中男性 1 617 例，女性 1 026 例，城区 1 706 例，郊区 937 例。男性世标发病率为女性的 1.68 倍，郊区世标发病率为城区的 1.01 倍。0~74 岁累积发病率为 1.12%（表 5.5.5）。

There were 2,643 new cases diagnosed as rectal cancer (C19-20; 1,617 males and 1,026 females, 1,706 in urban areas and 937 in peri-urban areas), accounting for 5.28% of new cases of all cancers in 2017. The crude incidence rate was 19.42 per 100,000, with an ASR China and an ASR World of 9.16 and 9.17 per 100,000, respectively. The incidence of ASR World was 68% higher in males than in females and 1% higher in peri-urban areas than in urban areas. The cumulative incidence rate for subjects aged 0 to 74 years was 1.12% (Table 5.5.5).

表 5.5.5 2017 年北京市户籍居民直肠癌（C19-20）发病情况
Table 5.5.5 Incidence of rectal cancer (C19-20) in Beijing, 2017

地区 Areas	性别 Sex	例数 No. cases	粗率 Crude rate （1/10⁵）	构成比 Freq.（%）	中标率 ASR China （1/10⁵）	世标率 ASR World （1/10⁵）	累积率 Cumulative rate(0~74, %)
全市 All areas	合计 Both	2 643	19.42	5.28	9.16	9.17	1.12
	男性 Male	1 617	23.81	6.53	11.47	11.59	1.44
	女性 Female	1 026	15.05	4.05	6.99	6.88	0.81
城区 Urban areas	合计 Both	1 706	20.21	5.17	9.11	9.14	1.11
	男性 Male	1 061	25.20	6.58	11.56	11.70	1.46
	女性 Female	645	15.25	3.82	6.80	6.71	0.78
郊区 Peri-urban areas	合计 Both	937	18.12	5.49	9.28	9.27	1.12
	男性 Male	556	21.54	6.44	11.33	11.46	1.41
	女性 Female	381	14.72	4.52	7.36	7.23	0.86

2017 年，北京市直肠癌（C19-20）死亡病例数为 1 255 例，占全部恶性肿瘤死亡的 4.82%，死亡率为 9.22/10 万，中标死亡率为 3.62/10 万，世标死亡率为 3.59/10 万；其中男性 773 例，女性 482 例，城区 833 例，郊区 422 例。男性世标死亡率为女性的 1.88 倍，郊区世标死亡率为城区的 1.09 倍。0~74 岁累积死亡率为 0.36%（表 5.5.6）。

A total of 1,255 cases died of rectal cancer (C19-20; 773 males and 482 females, 833 in urban areas and 422 in peri-urban areas), accounting for 4.82% of all cancer deaths in 2017. The crude mortality rate was 9.22 per 100,000, with an ASR China and an ASR World of 3.62 and 3.59 per 100,000, respectively. The mortality of ASR World was 88% higher in males than in females and 9% higher in peri-urban areas than in urban areas. The cumulative mortality rate for subjects aged 0 to 74 years was 0.36% (Table 5.5.6).

表 5.5.6 2017 年北京市户籍居民直肠癌（C19-20）死亡情况
Table 5.5.6 Mortality of rectal cancer(C19-20) in Beijing, 2017

地区 Areas	性别 Sex	例数 No. deaths	粗率 Crude rate $(1/10^5)$	构成比 Freq.（%）	中标率 ASR China $(1/10^5)$	世标率 ASR World $(1/10^5)$	累积率 Cumulative rate(0~74, %)
全市 All areas	合计 Both	1 255	9.22	4.82	3.62	3.59	0.36
	男性 Male	773	11.38	4.99	4.78	4.74	0.49
	女性 Female	482	7.07	4.57	2.55	2.53	0.23
城区 Urban areas	合计 Both	833	9.87	4.90	3.51	3.50	0.35
	男性 Male	534	12.69	5.35	4.82	4.79	0.49
	女性 Female	299	7.07	4.27	2.30	2.29	0.22
郊区 Peri-urban areas	合计 Both	422	8.16	4.66	3.86	3.81	0.37
	男性 Male	239	9.26	4.33	4.68	4.63	0.50
	女性 Female	183	7.07	5.17	3.09	3.04	0.25

北京市结直肠癌世标发病率由 2008 年的 17.02/10 万上升到 2017 年的 21.10/10 万，年均变化百分比为 2.45%（ $P<0.001$ ）；男性和女性发病 10 年间年均变化百分比分别为 3.24%（ $P<0.001$ ）和 1.38%（ $P=0.003$ ）。北京市结直肠癌世标死亡率由 2008 年的 7.64/10 万上升到 2017 年的 8.40/10 万，年均变化百分比为 0.63%（ $P=0.060$ ）；男性和女性死亡 10 年间年均变化百分比分别为 1.59%（ $P=0.005$ ）和 -0.66%（ $P=0.087$ ）。

结直肠癌年龄别发病率和死亡率在男性和女性中均随年龄呈上升趋势：发病率从 40~44 岁组之后上升明显，至 80~84 岁年龄组达高峰；年龄别死亡率从 40~44 岁组之后开始持续上升（图 5.5.1 至图 5.5.6）。45 岁以上年龄组男性各年龄别发病率和死亡率均明显高于女性（图 5.5.1 和图 5.5.4）。城区和郊区年龄别发病率、死亡率变化有一定差别，但总体趋势相同（图 5.5.2 和图 5.5.3，图 5.5.5 和图 5.5.6）。

The incidence of ASR World of colorectal cancer increased from 17.02 per 100,000 in 2008 to 21.10 per 100,000 in 2017; the APC of ASR World for incidence was 2.45% ($P<0.001$). The APCs of ASR World for incidence of colorectal cancer in males and females were 3.24% ($P<0.001$) and 1.38% ($P=0.003$), respectively. The mortality of ASR World of colorectal cancer increased from 7.64 per 100,000 in 2008 to 8.40 per 100,000 in 2017; the APC of ASR World for mortality was 0.63% ($P=0.060$). The APCs of ASR World for mortality of colorectal cancer in males and females were 1.59% ($P=0.005$) and -0.66% ($P=0.087$), respectively.

Trends of age-specific incidence and mortality rates of colorectal cancer were similar for males and females: the incidence rates for both sexes increased rapidly, starting with the age group of 40-44 years, and peaked at the age group of 80-84 years; and the mortality rates increased consistently, starting with the age group of 40-44 years (Figure 5.5.1-5.5.6). Age-specific incidence and mortality rates were consistently higher in males than in females, starting from the 45 years old age group (Figure 5.5.1, Figure 5.5.4). There were some differences in age-specific incidence and mortality rates between urban and peri-urban areas, but the overall trends were the same (Figure 5.5.2-5.5.3, Figure 5.5.5-5.5.6).

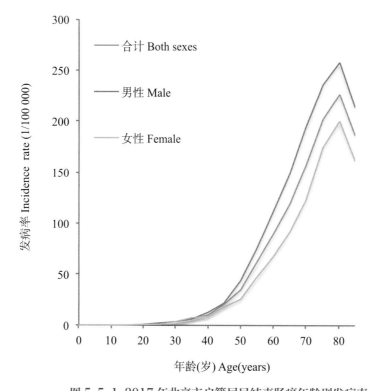

图 5.5.1 2017 年北京市户籍居民结直肠癌年龄别发病率

Figure 5.5.1 Age-specific incidence rates of colorectal cancer in Beijing, 2017

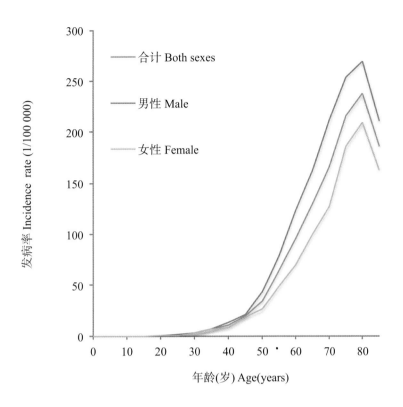

图 5.5.2 2017 年北京市城区户籍居民结直肠癌年龄别发病率
Figure 5.5.2 Age-specific incidence rates of colorectal cancer in urban areas of Beijing, 2017

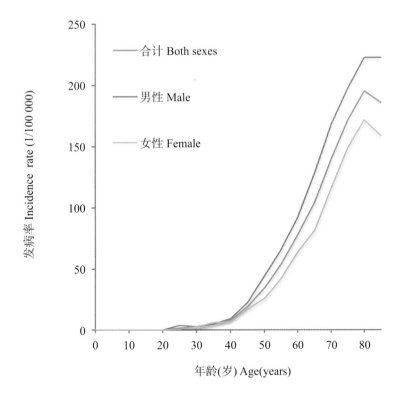

图 5.5.3 2017 年北京市郊区户籍居民结直肠癌年龄别发病率
Figure 5.5.3 Age-specific incidence rates of colorectal cancer in peri-urban areas of Beijing, 2017

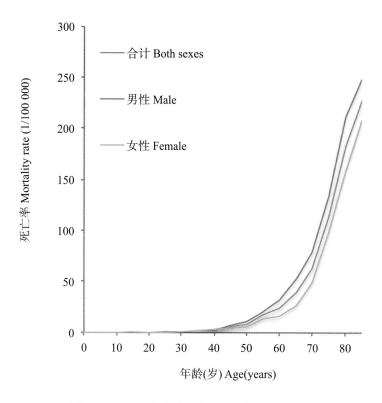

图 5.5.4 2017 年北京市户籍居民结直肠癌年龄别死亡率
Figure 5.5.4 Age-specific mortality rates of colorectal cancer in Beijing, 2017

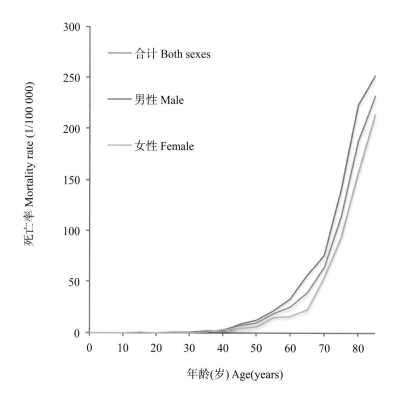

图 5.5.5 2017 年北京市城区户籍居民结直肠癌年龄别死亡率
Figure 5.5.5 Age-specific mortality rates of colorectal cancer in urban areas of Beijing, 2017

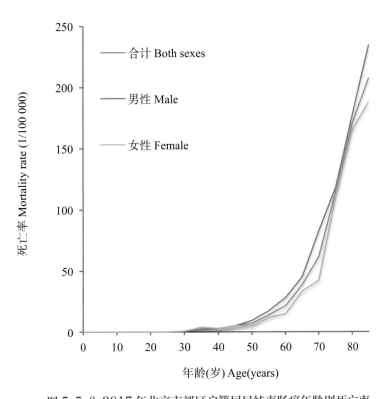

图 5.5.6 2017 年北京市郊区户籍居民结直肠癌年龄别死亡率
Figure 5.5.6 Age-specific mortality rates of colorectal cancer in peri-urban areas of Beijing, 2017

2017 年，北京市结直肠癌世标发病率和死亡率在 16 个辖区间存在一定差异，城区发病率和死亡率均高于郊区（图 5.5.7 和图 5.5.8）。

In 2017, there were some differences between the 16 districts in ASR World for incidence and mortality of colorectal cancer in Beijing. The incidence and mortality rates were both higher in urban areas than in peri-urban areas (Figure 5.5.7-5.5.8).

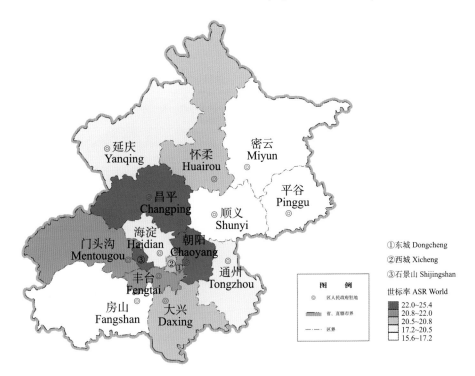

图 5.5.7 2017 年北京市户籍居民结直肠癌发病率（1/10⁵）地区分布情况
Figure 5.5.7 Incidence rates of colorectal cancer by district in Beijing, 2017 (1/10⁵)

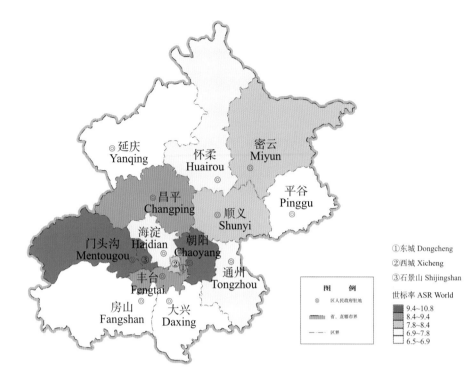

图 5.5.8　2017 年北京市户籍居民结直肠癌死亡率（1/10⁵）地区分布情况
Figure 5.5.8 Mortality rates of colorectal cancer by district in Beijing, 2017 $(1/10^5)$

全部结肠癌（C18）新发病例中，有明确亚部位的病例数占 73.86%。其中乙状结肠是最常见的发病部位，占 43.70%；其后依次为升结肠、降结肠和横结肠，分别占 25.02%、7.58% 和 6.91%（图 5.5.9）。

About 73.86% cases were assigned to specified categories of colon cancer (C18) site. Among those, sigmoid colon was the most common site, accounting for 43.70% of all cases, followed by the ascending colon (25.02%), the descending colon (7.58%) and the transverse colon (6.91%) (Figure 5.5.9).

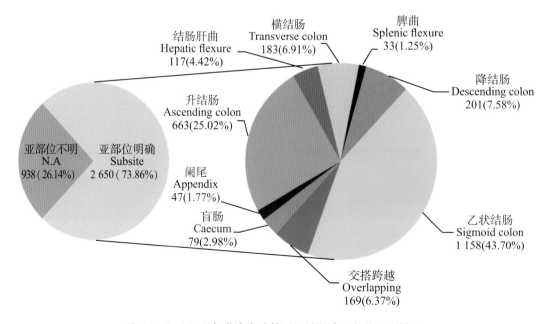

图 5.5.9　2017 年北京市户籍居民结肠癌亚部位分布情况
Figure 5.5.9 Subsite distribution of colon cancer in Beijing, 2017

（撰稿　张希，校稿　李晴雨）

5.6 肝 (C22)

5.6 Liver (C22)

2017 年，北京市肝癌新发病例数为 2 364 例，占全部恶性肿瘤发病的 4.72%，位居恶性肿瘤发病第 8 位；其中男性 1 670 例，女性 694 例，城区 1 467 例，郊区 897 例。肝癌发病率为 17.37/10 万，中标发病率为 8.39/10 万，世标发病率为 8.38/10 万；男性世标发病率为女性的 2.91 倍，郊区世标发病率为城区的 1.18 倍。0~74 岁累积发病率为 0.94%（表 5.6.1）。

There were 2,364 new cases diagnosed as liver cancer (1,670 males and 694 females, 1,467 in urban areas and 897 in peri-urban areas), accounting for 4.72% of new cases of all cancers in 2017. Liver cancer was the 8th common cancer in Beijing. The crude incidence rate was 17.37 per 100,000, with an ASR China and an ASR World of 8.39 and 8.38 per 100,000, respectively. The ASR World for incidence was 191% higher in males than in females and and 18% higher in peri-urban areas than in urban areas. The cumulative incidence rate for subjects aged 0 to 74 years was 0.94% (Table 5.6.1).

表 5.6.1 2017 年北京市户籍居民肝癌发病情况
Table 5.6.1 Incidence of liver cancer in Beijing, 2017

地区 Areas	性别 Sex	例数 No. cases	粗率 Crude rate (1/10^5)	构成比 Freq.（%）	中标率 ASR China (1/10^5)	世标率 ASR World (1/10^5)	累积率 Cumulative rate(0~74, %)	顺位 Rank
全市 All areas	合计 Both	2 364	17.37	4.72	8.39	8.38	0.94	8
	男性 Male	1 670	24.59	6.75	12.55	12.54	1.43	3
	女性 Female	694	10.18	2.74	4.32	4.31	0.46	9
城区 Urban areas	合计 Both	1 467	17.38	4.45	7.78	7.83	0.86	8
	男性 Male	1 021	24.25	6.34	11.60	11.64	1.31	5
	女性 Female	446	10.54	2.64	4.03	4.07	0.43	10
郊区 Peri-urban areas	合计 Both	897	17.35	5.25	9.31	9.24	1.06	6
	男性 Male	649	25.14	7.51	14.03	14.01	1.63	3
	女性 Female	248	9.58	2.94	4.76	4.68	0.52	9

2017 年，北京市肝癌死亡病例数为 2 249 例，占全部恶性肿瘤死亡的 8.63%，位居恶性肿瘤死亡第 3 位；其中男性 1 614 例，女性 635 例，城区 1 377 例，郊区 872 例。肝癌死亡率为 16.52/10 万，中标死亡率为 7.57/10 万，世标死亡率为 7.53/10 万；男性世标死亡率为女性的 3.24 倍，郊区世标死亡率为城区的 1.29 倍。0~74 岁累积死亡率为 0.84%（表 5.6.2）。

A total of 2,249 cases died of liver cancer (1,614 males and 635 females, 1,377 in urban areas and 872 in peri-urban areas), accounting for 8.63% of all cancer deaths in 2017. Liver cancer was the 3rd leading cause of cancer deaths in all cancers. The crude mortality rate was 16.52 per 100,000, with an ASR China and an ASR World of 7.57 and 7.53 per 100,000, respectively. The ASR World for mortality was 224% higher in males than in females and 29% higher in peri-urban areas than in urban areas, respectively. The cumulative mortality rate for subjects aged 0 to 74 years was 0.84% (Table 5.6.2).

表 5.6.2 2017 年北京市户籍居民肝癌死亡情况
Table 5.6.2 Mortality of liver cancer in Beijing, 2017

地区 Areas	性别 Sex	例数 No. deaths	粗率 Crude rate (1/10⁵)	构成比 Freq.（%）	中标率 ASR China (1/10⁵)	世标率 ASR World (1/10⁵)	累积率 Cumulative rate(0~74,%)	顺位 Rank
全市 All areas	合计 Both	2 249	16.52	8.63	7.57	7.53	0.84	3
	男性 Male	1 614	23.77	10.41	11.63	11.60	1.31	3
	女性 Female	635	9.31	6.02	3.63	3.58	0.38	4
城区 Urban areas	合计 Both	1 377	16.31	8.11	6.81	6.79	0.73	4
	男性 Male	977	23.21	9.79	10.54	10.50	1.16	3
	女性 Female	400	9.46	5.71	3.17	3.16	0.31	4
郊区 Peri-urban areas	合计 Both	872	16.87	9.62	8.77	8.72	1.01	2
	男性 Male	637	24.67	11.54	13.38	13.42	1.56	2
	女性 Female	235	9.08	6.63	4.33	4.23	0.49	4

北京市肝癌世标发病率由 2008 年的 13.01/10 万下降到 2017 年的 8.38/10 万，年均变化百分比为 -4.27%（P<0.001）；男性和女性发病 10 年间年均变化百分比分别为 -4.28%（P<0.001）和 -4.40%（P<0.001）。北京市肝癌世标死亡率由 2008 年的 10.30/10 万下降到 2017 年的 7.53/10 万，年均变化百分比为 -3.73%（P<0.001）；男性和女性死亡 10 年间年均变化百分比分别为 -3.59%（P<0.001）和 -4.29%（P<0.001）。

肝癌年龄别发病率和死亡率呈现明显性别差异，除低年龄组略有波动外，35 岁以上各年龄组，男性发病率与死亡率均高于女性。无论男女，肝癌年龄别发病率和死亡率在 0 岁组有一个小高峰，30 岁之前整体处于较低水平，30 岁之后开始快速升高。男性发病和死亡分别在 85 岁及以上年龄组和

The ASR World for incidence of liver cancer decreased from 13.01 per 100,000 in 2008 to 8.38 per 100,000 in 2017; the APC of ASR World for incidence of was −4.27% (P<0.001) .The APCs of ASR World for incidence of liver cancer in males and females were −4.28% (P<0.001) and −4.40% (P<0.001), respectively. The ASR World for mortality of liver cancer decreased from 10.30 per 100,000 in 2008 to 7.53 per 100,000 in 2017; the APC of ASR World for mortality was −3.73% (P<0.001). The APCs of ASR World for mortality of liver cancer in males and females were −3.59% (P<0.001) and −4.29% (P<0.001), respectively.

The trends of age-specific incidence and mortality rates showed differences between males and females in Beijing. Except for the slight fluctuation observed in lower age groups, age-specific incidence and mortality rates of liver cancers were consistently higher in males than in females starting from the age group of 30-40 years old. The age-specific incidence and mortality rates for both sexes had a smaller peak in the age group of 0 year old. Both age-specific incidence and mortality rates were relatively low in people aged below 30 years old and increased sharply thereafter. The incidence and mortality rates for males peaked at the

80~84 岁组达到高峰；女性发病在 80~84 岁组达到高峰，死亡在 85 岁及以上年龄组达到高峰（图 5.6.1 至图 5.6.6）。

age group of 85 years and above and 80~84 years, respectively, and those for females peaked at the age group of 80~84 years and 85 years and above, respectively (Figure 5.6.1-5.6.6).

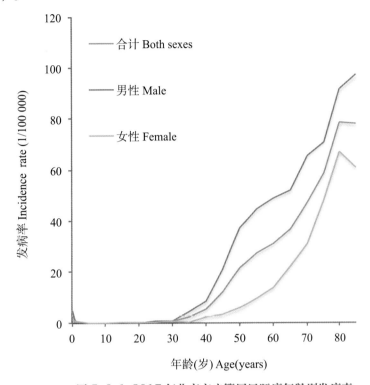

图 5.6.1 2017 年北京市户籍居民肝癌年龄别发病率

Figure 5.6.1 Age-specific incidence rates of liver cancer in Beijing, 2017

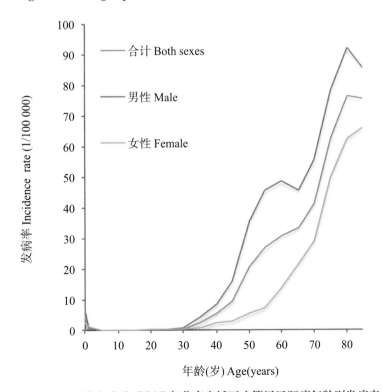

图 5.6.2 2017 年北京市城区户籍居民肝癌年龄别发病率

Figure 5.6.2 Age-specific incidence rates of liver cancer in urban areas of Beijing, 2017

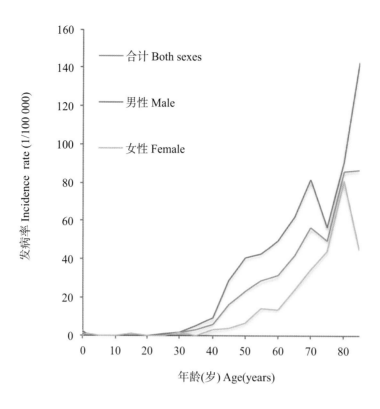

图 5.6.3 2017 年北京市郊区户籍居民肝癌年龄别发病率

Figure 5.6.3 Age-specific incidence rates of liver cancer in peri-urban areas of Beijing, 2017

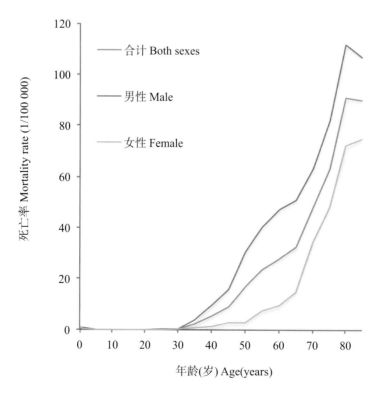

图 5.6.4 2017 年北京市户籍居民肝癌年龄别死亡率

Figure 5.6.4 Age-specific mortality rates of liver cancer in Beijing, 2017

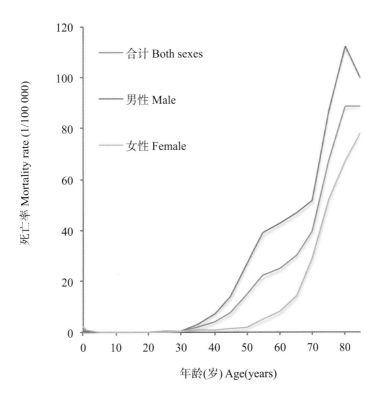

图 5.6.5　2017 年北京市城区户籍居民肝癌年龄别死亡率

Figure 5.6.5 Age-specific mortality rates of liver cancer in urban areas of Beijing, 2017

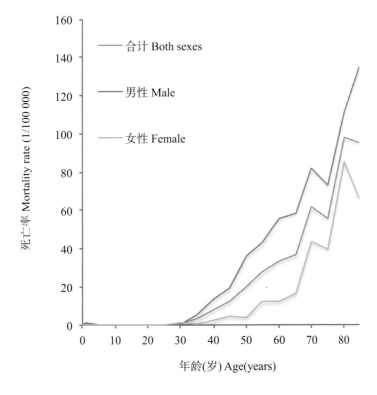

图 5.6.6　2017 年北京市郊区户籍居民肝癌年龄别死亡率

Figure 5.6.6 Age-specific mortality rates of liver cancer in peri-urban areas of Beijing, 2017

2017年，北京市肝癌世标发病率和死亡率在16个辖区间有一定差异，郊区发病率和死亡率均高于城区（图5.6.7和图5.6.8）。

In 2017, there were some differences between the 16 districts in ASR World for incidence and mortality of liver cancer in Beijing. The incidence and mortality rates were higher in peri-urban areas than in urban areas（Figure 5.6.7-5.6.8）.

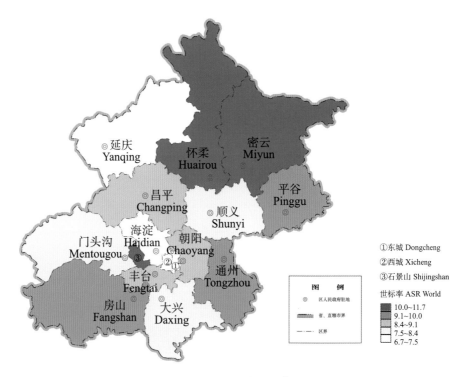

图 5.6.7　2017 年北京市户籍居民肝癌发病率（1/10^5）地区分布情况

Figure 5.6.7　Incidence rates of liver cancer by district in Beijing, 2017(1/10^5)

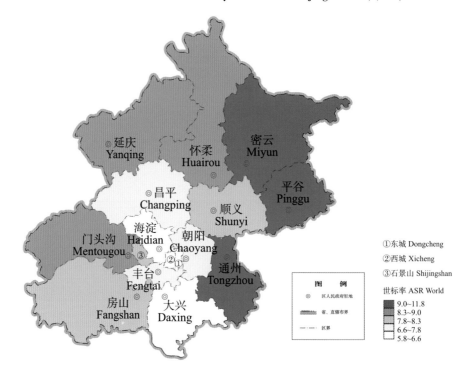

图 5.6.8　2017 年北京市户籍居民肝癌死亡率（1/10^5）地区分布情况

Figure 5.6.8　Mortality rates of liver cancer by district in Beijing, 2017(1/10^5)

（撰稿　李慧超，校稿　刘硕）

5.7 胆囊 (C23-24)

　　2017年,北京市胆囊癌新发病例数为1 085例,占全部恶性肿瘤发病的2.17%,位居恶性肿瘤发病第17位;其中男性572例,女性513例,城区651例,郊区434例。胆囊癌发病率为7.97/10万,中标发病率为3.44/10万,世标发病率为3.39/10万;男性世标发病率为女性的1.26倍,郊区世标发病率为城区的1.33倍。0~74岁累积发病率为0.40%(表5.7.1)。

5.7 Gallbladder (C23-24)

　　There were 1,085 new cases diagnosed as gallbladder cancer (572 males and 513 females, 651 in urban areas and 434 in peri-urban areas), accounting for 2.17% of new cases of all cancers in 2017. Gallbladder cancer was the 17th common cancer in Beijing. The crude incidence rate was 7.97 per 100,000, with an ASR China and an ASR World of 3.44 and 3.39 per 100,000, respectively. The ASR World for incidence was 26% higher in males than in females and 33% higher in peri-urban areas than in urban areas. The cumulative incidence rate for subjects aged 0 to 74 years was 0.40% (Table 5.7.1).

表 5.7.1　2017 年北京市户籍居民胆囊癌发病情况
Table 5.7.1 Incidence of gallbladder cancer in Beijing, 2017

地区 Areas	性别 Sex	例数 No. cases	粗率 Crude rate (1/10^5)	构成比 Freq.(%)	中标率 ASR China (1/10^5)	世标率 ASR World (1/10^5)	累积率 Cumulative rate(0~74, %)	顺位 Rank
全市 All areas	合计 Both	1 085	7.97	2.17	3.44	3.39	0.40	17
	男性 Male	572	8.42	2.31	3.83	3.80	0.45	13
	女性 Female	513	7.52	2.03	3.08	3.01	0.35	14
城区 Urban areas	合计 Both	651	7.71	1.97	3.08	3.03	0.35	17
	男性 Male	333	7.91	2.07	3.44	3.40	0.40	13
	女性 Female	318	7.52	1.88	2.73	2.68	0.30	14
郊区 Peri-urban areas	合计 Both	434	8.39	2.54	4.11	4.05	0.48	17
	男性 Male	239	9.26	2.77	4.64	4.61	0.53	13
	女性 Female	195	7.53	2.31	3.62	3.53	0.43	12

2017 年，北京市胆囊癌死亡病例数为 846 例，占全部恶性肿瘤死亡的 3.25%，位居恶性肿瘤死亡第 12 位；其中男性 452 例，女性 394 例，城区 490 例，郊区 356 例。胆囊癌死亡率为 6.22/10 万，中标死亡率为 2.50/10 万，世标死亡率为 2.46/10 万；男性世标死亡率为女性的 1.31 倍，郊区世标死亡率为城区的 1.56 倍。0~74 岁累积死亡率为 0.26%（表 5.7.2）。

A total of 846 cases died of gallbladder cancer (452 males and 394 females, 490 in urban areas and 356 in peri-urban areas), accounting for 3.25% of all cancer deaths in 2017. Gallbladder cancer was the 12th leading cause of cancer deaths in all cancers. The crude mortality rate was 6.22 per 100,000, with an ASR China and an ASR World of 2.50 and 2.46 per 100,000, respectively. The ASR World for mortality was 31% higher in males than in females and 56% higher in peri-urban areas than in urban areas. The cumulative mortality rate for subjects aged 0 to 74 years was 0.26% (Table 5.7.2).

表 5.7.2 2017 年北京市户籍居民胆囊癌死亡情况
Table 5.7.2 Mortality of gallbladder cancer in Beijing, 2017

地区 Areas	性别 Sex	例数 No. deaths	粗率 Crude rate （1/10^5）	构成比 Freq.（%）	中标率 ASR China （1/10^5）	世标率 ASR World （1/10^5）	累积率 Cumulative rate(0~74, %)	顺位 Rank
全市 All areas	合计 Both	846	6.22	3.25	2.50	2.46	0.26	12
	男性 Male	452	6.66	2.92	2.82	2.80	0.31	11
	女性 Female	394	5.78	3.74	2.21	2.14	0.21	9
城区 Urban areas	合计 Both	490	5.81	2.88	2.10	2.06	0.21	14
	男性 Male	252	5.99	2.52	2.30	2.30	0.26	12
	女性 Female	238	5.63	3.40	1.90	1.82	0.17	9
郊区 Peri-urban areas	合计 Both	356	6.89	3.93	3.28	3.21	0.33	8
	男性 Male	200	7.75	3.62	3.84	3.72	0.40	7
	女性 Female	156	6.03	4.40	2.76	2.73	0.28	7

北京市胆囊癌世标发病率由 2008 年的 3.17/10 万上升到 2017 年的 3.39/10 万，年均变化百分比为 0.12%（P=0.838）；男性和女性发病 10 年间年均变化百分比分别为 0.94%（P=0.066）和 -0.78%（P=0.352）。北京市胆囊癌世标死亡率由 2008 年的 2.66/10 万下降到 2017 年的 2.46/10 万，年均变化百分比为 -0.55%（P=0.423）；男性和女性死亡 10 年间年均变化百分比分别为 0.52%（P=0.320）和 -1.80%（P=0.158）。

胆囊癌年龄别发病率和死亡率在 40 岁以前均较低，40 岁以后快速上升，男性上升速度高于女性（图 5.7.1 至图 5.7.6）。除 50~54 岁年龄组女性发病率略高于男性，40~44 岁和 75~79 岁年龄组女性死亡率略高于男性外，40 岁以上年龄组男性胆囊癌发病率和死亡率均高于女性。男性和女性的发病率均在 80~84 岁年龄组达到高峰；男性死亡率在 80~84 岁年龄组达到高峰，女性死亡率在 85 岁及以上年龄组达到高峰（图 5.7.1 和图 5.7.4）。城区和郊区年龄别发病率、死亡率变化有一定差别，但总体趋势相同，郊区的发病率和死亡率始终高于城区（图 5.7.2 和图 5.7.3，图 5.7.5 和图 5.7.6）。

The incidence of ASR World of gallbladder cancer increased from 3.17 per 100,000 in 2008 to 3.39 per 100,000 in 2017; the APC of ASR World for incidence was 0.12 (P=0.838). The APCs of ASR World for incidence of gallbladder cancer in males and females were 0.94% (P=0.066) and -0.78% (P=0.352), respectively. The mortality of ASR World of gallbladder cancer decreased from 2.66 per 100,000 in 2008 to 2.46 per 100,000 in 2017; the APC of ASR World for mortality was -0.55% (P=0.423). The APCs of ASR World for mortality of gallbladder cancer in males and females were 0.52% (P=0.320) and -1.80% (P=0.158), respectively.

The age-specific incidence and mortality rates of gallbladder cancer were relatively low in people below 40 years old, and the rates increased sharply in people older than that, and the growth rates were higher in males than in females (Figure 5.7.1-5.7.6). Except the incidence rate at the age group of 50-54 years and the mortality rates at the age group of 40-44 and 75-79 years were slightly higher in females than those in males, the incidence and mortality rates in males were consistently higher than those in females after 40 years old. And the age-specific incidence and mortality rates for both sexes peaked at the age group of 80-84 years, except the age-specific mortality rates for females peaked at the age group of 85 years and above (Figure 5.7.1, Figure 5.7.4). There were some differences in age-specific incidence and mortality rates between urban and peri-urban areas, but the overall trends were same. The age-specific incidence and mortality rates in peri-urban areas were consistently higher than those in urban areas (Figure 5.7.2-5.7.3, Figure 5.7.5-5.7.6).

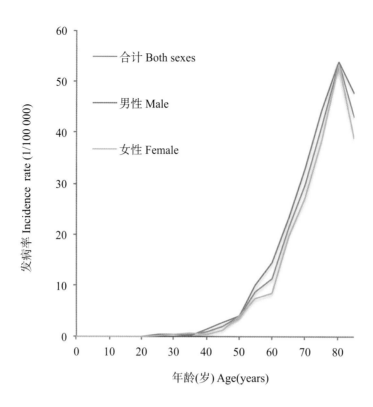

图 5.7.1 2017 年北京市户籍居民胆囊癌年龄别发病率
Figure 5.7.1 Age-specific incidence rates of gallbladder cancer in Beijing, 2017

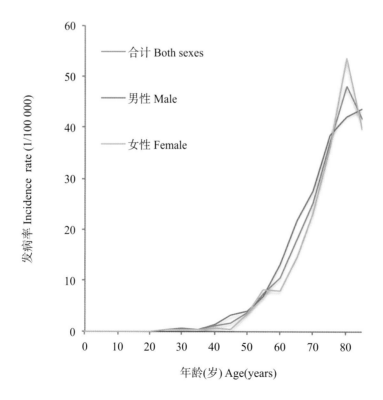

图 5.7.2 2017 年北京市城区户籍居民胆囊癌年龄别发病率
Figure 5.7.2 Age-specific incidence rates of gallbladder cancer in urban areas of Beijing, 2017

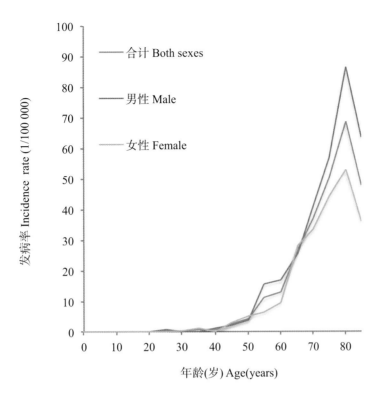

图 5.7.3 2017 年北京市郊区户籍居民胆囊癌年龄别发病率
Figure 5.7.3 Age-specific incidence rates of gallbladder cancer in peri-urban areas of Beijing, 2017

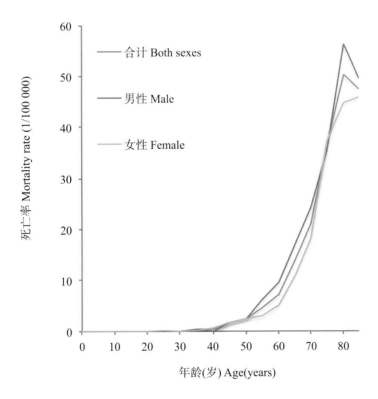

图 5.7.4 2017 年北京市户籍居民胆囊癌年龄别死亡率
Figure 5.7.4 Age-specific mortality rates of gallbladder cancer in Beijing, 2017

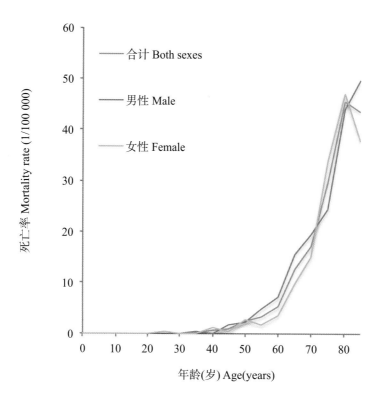

图 5.7.5 2017 年北京市城区户籍居民胆囊癌年龄别死亡率
Figure 5.7.5 Age-specific mortality rates of gallbladder cancer in urban areas of Beijing, 2017

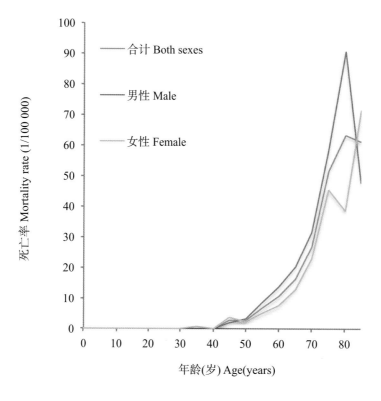

图 5.7.6 2017 年北京市郊区户籍居民胆囊癌年龄别死亡率
Figure 5.7.6 Age-specific mortality rates of gallbladder cancer in peri-urban areas of Beijing, 2017

（撰稿 张倩，校稿 李晴雨）

5.8 胰腺 (C25)

2017年,北京市胰腺癌新发病例数为1412例,占全部恶性肿瘤发病的2.82%,位居恶性肿瘤发病第13位;其中男性811例,女性601例,城区963例,郊区449例。胰腺癌发病率为10.37/10万,中标发病率为4.65/10万,世标发病率为4.58/10万;男性世标发病率为女性的1.61倍,城区世标发病率为郊区的1.10倍。0~74岁累积发病率为0.55%(表5.8.1)。

5.8 Pancreas (C25)

There were 1,412 new cases diagnosed as pancreatic cancer (811 males and 601 females, 963 in urban areas and 449 in peri-urban areas), accounting for 2.82% of new cases of all cancers in 2017. Pancreatic cancer was the 13th common cancer in Beijing. The crude incidence rate was 10.37 per 100,000, with an ASR China and an ASR World of 4.65 and 4.58 per 100,000, respectively. The ASR World for incidence was 61% higher in males than in females and 10% higher in urban areas than in peri-urban areas. The cumulative incidence rate for subjects aged 0 to 74 years was 0.55% (Table 5.8.1).

表 5.8.1 2017 年北京市户籍居民胰腺癌发病情况
Table 5.8.1 Incidence of pancreatic cancer in Beijing, 2017

地区 Areas	性别 Sex	例数 No. cases	粗率 Crude rate (1/10^5)	构成比 Freq.(%)	中标率 ASR China (1/10^5)	世标率 ASR World (1/10^5)	累积率 Cumulative rate(0~74,%)	顺位 Rank
全市 All areas	合计 Both	1 412	10.37	2.82	4.65	4.58	0.55	13
	男性 Male	811	11.94	3.28	5.77	5.68	0.71	11
	女性 Female	601	8.81	2.37	3.57	3.52	0.39	12
城区 Urban areas	合计 Both	963	11.41	2.92	4.79	4.73	0.55	13
	男性 Male	532	12.64	3.30	5.76	5.70	0.70	9
	女性 Female	431	10.19	2.55	3.83	3.78	0.41	11
郊区 Peri-urban areas	合计 Both	449	8.68	2.63	4.40	4.32	0.53	16
	男性 Male	279	10.81	3.23	5.80	5.66	0.73	11
	女性 Female	170	6.57	2.02	3.10	3.06	0.35	14

2017年,北京市胰腺癌死亡病例数为1 320例,占全部恶性肿瘤死亡的5.07%,位居恶性肿瘤死亡第6位;其中男性766例,女性554例,城区917例,郊区403例。胰腺癌死亡率为9.70/10万,中标死亡率为4.16/10万,世标死亡率为4.09/10万;男性世标死亡率为女性的1.68倍,城区世标死亡率为郊区的1.13倍。0~74岁累积死亡率为0.49%(表5.8.2)。

A total of 1,320 cases died of pancreatic cancer (766 males and 554 females, 917 in urban areas and 403 in peri-urban areas), accounting for 5.07% of all cancer deaths in 2017. Pancreatic cancer was the 6th leading cause of cancer deaths in all cancers. The crude mortality rate was 9.70 per 100,000, with an ASR China and an ASR World of 4.16 and 4.09 per 100,000, respectively. The ASR World for mortality was 68% higher in males than in females and 13% higher in urban areas than in peri-urban areas. The cumulative mortality rate for subjects aged 0 to 74 years was 0.49% (Table 5.8.2).

表 5.8.2 2017 年北京市户籍居民胰腺癌死亡情况
Table 5.8.2 Mortality of pancreatic cancer in Beijing, 2017

地区 Areas	性别 Sex	例数 No. deaths	粗率 Crude rate (1/10^5)	构成比 Freq.(%)	中标率 ASR China (1/10^5)	世标率 ASR World (1/10^5)	累积率 Cumulative rate(0~74,%)	顺位 Rank
全市 All areas	合计 Both	1 320	9.70	5.07	4.16	4.09	0.49	6
	男性 Male	766	11.28	4.94	5.27	5.18	0.66	6
	女性 Female	554	8.12	5.25	3.12	3.08	0.34	5
城区 Urban areas	合计 Both	917	10.86	5.40	4.30	4.27	0.51	6
	男性 Male	521	12.38	5.22	5.40	5.36	0.68	5
	女性 Female	396	9.36	5.65	3.26	3.24	0.35	5
郊区 Peri-urban areas	合计 Both	403	7.79	4.45	3.90	3.77	0.46	7
	男性 Male	245	9.49	4.44	5.04	4.86	0.63	6
	女性 Female	158	6.10	4.46	2.83	2.75	0.31	6

北京市胰腺癌世标发病率由2008年的4.62/10万下降到2017年的4.58/10万,年均变化百分比为0.00%(P=0.994);男性和女性发病10年间年均变化百分比分别为0.49%(P=0.319)和-0.69%(P=0.303)。北京市

The incidence of ASR World of pancreatic cancer decreased from 4.62 per 100,000 in 2008 to 4.58 per 100,000 in 2017; the APC of ASR World for incidence was 0.00% (P=0.994). The APCs of ASR World for incidence of pancreatic cancer in males and females were 0.49% (P=0.319) and -0.69% (P=0.303), respectively. The mortality of ASR World of pancreatic

胰腺癌世标死亡率由 2008 年的 3.62/10 万上升到 2017 年的 4.09/10 万，年均变化百分比为 0.64%（P=0.211）；男性和女性死亡 10 年间年均变化百分比分别为 1.21%（P=0.135）和 -0.16%（P=0.843）。

胰腺癌年龄别发病率和死亡率在 45 岁以前均较低，45 岁以后快速上升，发病率和死亡率均在 80~84 岁组达到高峰（图 5.8.1 至图 5.8.6）。除 85 岁及以上年龄组外，45 岁及以上年龄组男性胰腺癌发病率和死亡率均高于女性，男性和女性发病率分别在 80~84 岁和 85 岁及以上年龄组达到高峰，死亡率均在 80~84 岁年龄组达到高峰（图 5.8.1 和图 5.8.4）。城区和郊区年龄别发病率、死亡率变化有一定差别，但总体趋势相同，郊区波动较为明显（图 5.8.2 和图 5.8.3，图 5.8.5 和图 5.8.6）。

cancer increased from 3.62 per 100,000 in 2008 to 4.09 per 100,000 in 2017; the APC of ASR World for mortality was 0.64% (P=0.211). The APCs of ASR World for mortality of pancreatic cancer in males and females were 1.21% (P=0.135) and -0.16% (P=0.843), respectively.

The age-specific incidence and mortality rates of pancreatic cancer were relatively low in people below 45 years old, and the rates increased sharply in people older than that, furthermore, both the incidence and mortality rates peaked at the age group of 80-84 years age group (Figure 5.8.1-5.8.6). Except for the age group of 85 years and above, the incidence and mortality rates in males were consistently higher than those in females after 45 years old. And the age-specific incidence rates for males and females peaked at the age group of 80-84 years and the age group of 85 years and above, respectively, and the age-specific mortality rates for both sexes peaked at the age group of 80-84 years (Figure 5.8.1, Figure 5.8.4). There were some differences in age-specific incidence and mortality rates between urban and peri-urban areas, but the overall trends were same. The age-specific incidence and mortality rates in peri-urban areas showed significant fluctuations (Figure 5.8.2-5.8.3, Figure 5.8.5-5.8.6).

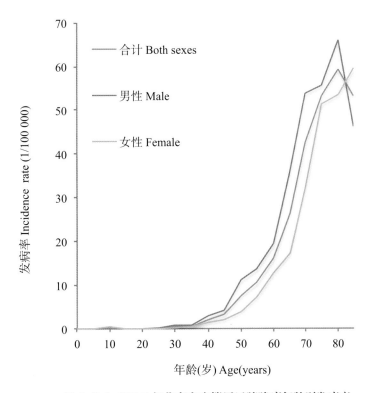

图 5.8.1 2017 年北京市户籍居民胰腺癌年龄别发病率
Figure 5.8.1 Age-specific incidence rates of pancreatic cancer in Beijing, 2017

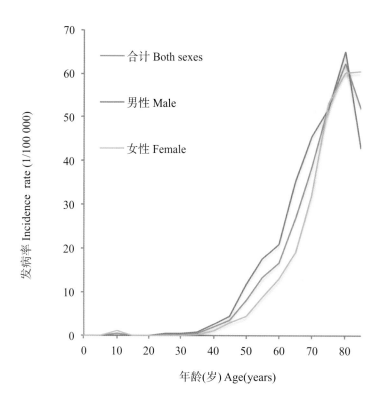

图 5.8.2 2017 年北京市城区户籍居民胰腺癌年龄别发病率
Figure 5.8.2 Age-specific incidence rates of pancreatic cancer in urban areas of Beijing, 2017

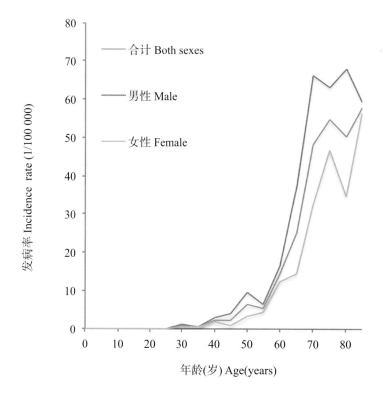

图 5.8.3 2017 年北京市郊区户籍居民胰腺癌年龄别发病率
Figure 5.8.3 Age-specific incidence rates of pancreatic cancer in peri-urban areas of Beijing, 2017

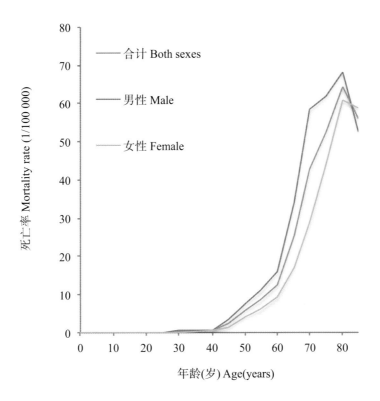

图 5.8.4 2017 年北京市户籍居民胰腺癌年龄别死亡率
Figure 5.8.4 Age-specific mortality rates of pancreatic cancer in Beijing, 2017

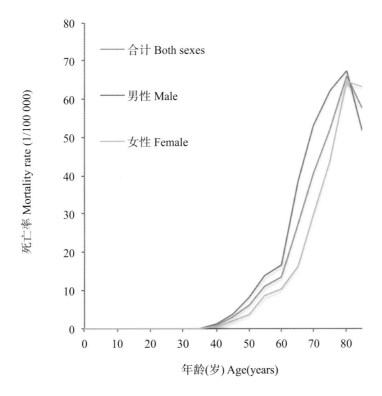

图 5.8.5 2017 年北京市城区户籍居民胰腺癌年龄别死亡率
Figure 5.8.5 Age-specific mortality rates of pancreatic cancer in urban areas of Beijing, 2017

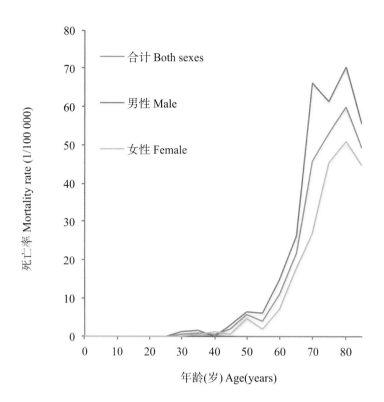

图 5.8.6 2017 年北京市郊区户籍居民胰腺癌年龄别死亡率

Figure 5.8.6 Age-specific mortality rates of pancreatic cancer in peri-urban areas of Beijing, 2017

全部胰腺癌新发病例中，有明确亚部位的病例数占 24.01%，其中胰头是最常见的发病部位，占 56.64%；其后依次为胰岛（朗格汉斯岛）、胰尾、胰体，分别占 15.93%、11.50% 和 10.03%（图 5.8.7）。

About 24.01% cases were assigned to specified categories of pancreatic cancer site. Among those, head of pancreas was the most common subsite, accounting for 56.64% of all cases, followed by the islets of Langerhans (15.93%), the tail (11.50%) and the body (10.03%) (Figure 5.8.7).

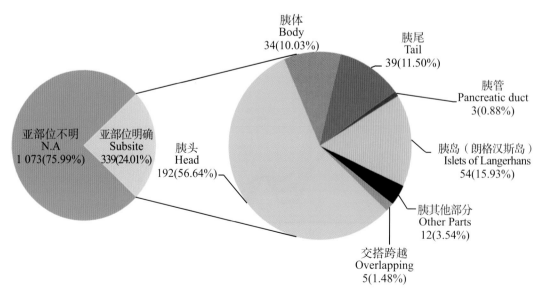

图 5.8.7 2017 年北京市户籍居民胰腺癌亚部位分布情况

Figure 5.8.7 Subsite distribution of pancreatic cancer in Beijing, 2017

（撰稿 张倩，校稿 李晴雨）

5.9 喉 (C32)

　　2017 年，北京市喉癌新发病例数为 291 例，占全部恶性肿瘤发病的 0.58%，位居恶性肿瘤发病第 20 位；其中男性 274 例，女性 17 例，城区 175 例，郊区 116 例。喉癌发病率为 2.14/10 万，中标发病率为 1.02/10 万，世标发病率为 1.04/10 万；男性世标发病率为女性的 22.31 倍，郊区世标发病率为城区的 1.16 倍。0~74 岁累积发病率为 0.13%（表 5.9.1）。

5.9 Larynx (C32)

　　There were 291 new cases diagnosed as larynx cancer (274 males and 17 females, 175 in urban areas and 116 in peri-urban areas), accounting for 0.58% of new cases of all cancers in 2017. Larynx cancer was the 20th common cancer in Beijing. The crude incidence rate was 2.14 per 100,000, with an ASR China and an ASR World of 1.02 and 1.04 per 100,000, respectively. The ASR World for incidence was 2131% higher in males than in females and 16% higher in peri-urban areas than in urban areas. The cumulative incidence rate for subjects aged 0 to 74 years was 0.13% (Table 5.9.1).

表 5.9.1 2017 年北京市户籍居民喉癌发病情况
Table 5.9.1 Incidence of larynx cancer in Beijing, 2017

地区 Areas	性别 Sex	例数 No. cases	粗率 Crude rate (1/10^5)	构成比 Freq.（%）	中标率 ASR China (1/10^5)	世标率 ASR World (1/10^5)	累积率 Cumulative rate(0~74, %)	顺位 Rank
全市 All areas	合计 Both	291	2.14	0.58	1.02	1.04	0.13	20
	男性 Male	274	4.03	1.11	1.99	2.03	0.25	16
	女性 Female	17	0.25	0.07	0.09	0.09	0.01	23
城区 Urban areas	合计 Both	175	2.07	0.53	0.95	0.98	0.12	20
	男性 Male	163	3.87	1.01	1.84	1.90	0.23	16
	女性 Female	12	0.28	0.07	0.10	0.10	0.01	23
郊区 Peri-urban areas	合计 Both	116	2.24	0.68	1.14	1.14	0.14	20
	男性 Male	111	4.30	1.28	2.27	2.25	0.28	16
	女性 Female	5	0.19	0.06	0.08	0.08	0.01	23

2017 年，北京市喉癌死亡病例数为 126 例，占全部恶性肿瘤死亡的 0.48%，位居恶性肿瘤死亡第 19 位；其中男性 113 例，女性 13 例，城区 70 例，郊区 56 例。喉癌死亡率为 0.93/10 万，中标死亡率为 0.36/10 万，世标死亡率为 0.36/10 万；男性世标死亡率为女性的 14.79 倍，郊区世标死亡率为城区的 1.71 倍。0~74 岁累积死亡率为 0.04%（表 5.9.2）。

A total of 126 cases died of larynx cancer (113 males and 13 females, 70 in urban areas and 56 in peri-urban areas), accounting for 0.48% of all cancer deaths in 2017. Larynx cancer was the 19th leading cause of cancer deaths in all cancers. The crude mortality rate was 0.93 per 100,000, with an ASR China and an ASR World of both 0.36 per 100,000. The ASR World for mortality was 1379% higher in males than in females and 71% higher in peri-urban areas than in urban areas, respectively. The cumulative mortality rate for subjects aged 0 to 74 years was 0.04% (Table 5.9.2).

表 5.9.2 2017 年北京市户籍居民喉癌死亡情况
Table 5.9.2 Mortality of larynx cancer in Beijing, 2017

地区 Areas	性别 Sex	例数 No. deaths	粗率 Crude rate (1/10^5)	构成比 Freq.(%)	中标率 ASR China (1/10^5)	世标率 ASR World (1/10^5)	累积率 Cumulative rate(0~74, %)	顺位 Rank
全市 All areas	合计 Both	126	0.93	0.48	0.36	0.36	0.04	19
	男性 Male	113	1.66	0.73	0.70	0.70	0.08	15
	女性 Female	13	0.19	0.12	0.05	0.05	0.00	23
城区 Urban areas	合计 Both	70	0.83	0.41	0.29	0.29	0.03	21
	男性 Male	61	1.45	0.61	0.55	0.55	0.06	15
	女性 Female	9	0.21	0.13	0.05	0.05	0.00	23
郊区 Peri-urban areas	合计 Both	56	1.08	0.62	0.50	0.50	0.05	20
	男性 Male	52	2.01	0.94	0.99	0.98	0.11	15
	女性 Female	4	0.15	0.11	0.05	0.05	—	23

北京市喉癌世标发病率由 2008 年的 1.07/10 万下降到 2017 年的 1.04/10 万，年均变化百分比为 -0.21%（P=0.717）；男性和女性发病 10 年间年均变化百分比分别为 0.08%（P=0.888）和 -5.27%（P=0.037）。北京市喉癌世标死亡率由 2008 年的 0.45/10 万下降到 2017 年的 0.36/10 万，年均变化百分比为 -2.08%（P=0.194）；男性和女性死亡 10 年间年均变化百分比分别为 -1.51%（P=0.330）和 -7.08%（P=0.047）。

喉癌年龄别发病率和死亡率在 45 岁以前均较低，45 岁以后快速上升，男性上升速度高于女性（图 5.9.1 至图 5.9.6）。整个年龄周期总体呈现男性喉癌发病率和死亡率高于女性，男性和女性发病率均在 75~79 岁年龄组达到高峰，死亡率均在 80~84 岁年龄组达到高峰（图 5.9.1 和图 5.9.4）。城区年龄别发病率呈现"双峰"特征，60~64 岁组出现一个高峰，在 75~79 岁组达到另一个高峰；郊区年龄别发病率在 75~79 岁组达到高峰。城区和郊区年龄别死亡率变化有一定差别，但总体趋势相同（图 5.9.2 和图 5.9.3，图 5.9.5 和图 5.9.6）。

The incidence of ASR World of larynx cancer decreased from 1.07 per 100,000 in 2008 to 1.04 per 100,000 in 2017; the APC of ASR World for incidence was -0.21% (P=0.717). The APCs of ASR World for incidence of larynx cancer in males and females were 0.08% (P=0.888) and -5.27% (P=0.037), respectively. The mortality of ASR World of larynx cancer decreased from 0.45 per 100,000 in 2008 to 0.36 per 100,000 in 2017; the APC of ASR World for mortality was -2.08% (P=0.194). The APCs of ASR World for mortality of larynx cancer in males and females were -1.51% (P=0.330) and -7.08% (P=0.047), respectively.

The age-specific incidence and mortality rates of larynx cancer were relatively low in people below 45 years old, and the rates increased sharply in people older than that, and the growth rates were higher in males than in females (Figure 5.9.1-5.9.6). The incidence and mortality rates in males were consistently higher than in females across all age groups. And the age-specific incidence rates for both males and females peaked at the age group of 75-79 years, and the age-specific mortality rates for both sexes peaked at the age group of 80-84 years (Figure 5.9.1, Figure 5.9.4). The age-specific incidence rates of larynx cancer in urban areas showed a double-peak phenomenon. The first peak appeared at the age of 60-64 years old and the second peak appeared at the age of 75-79 years old. The age-specific incidence rates of larynx cancer in peri-urban areas reached peak at the age of 75-79 years old. There were some differences in age-specific mortality rates between urban and peri-urban areas, but the overall trends were same (Figure 5.9.2-5.9.3, Figure 5.9.5-5.9.6).

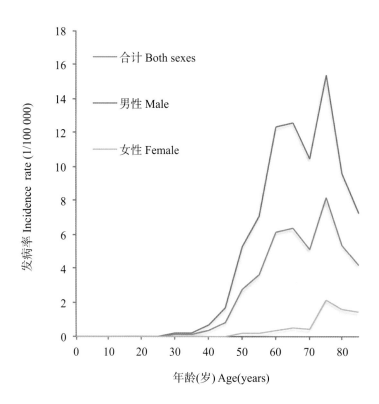

图 5.9.1 2017 年北京市户籍居民喉癌年龄别发病率

Figure 5.9.1 Age-specific incidence rates of larynx cancer in Beijing, 2017

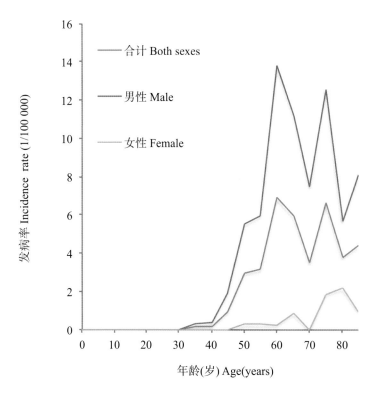

图 5.9.2 2017 年北京市城区户籍居民喉癌年龄别发病率

Figure 5.9.2 Age-specific incidence rates of larynx cancer in urban areas of Beijing, 2017

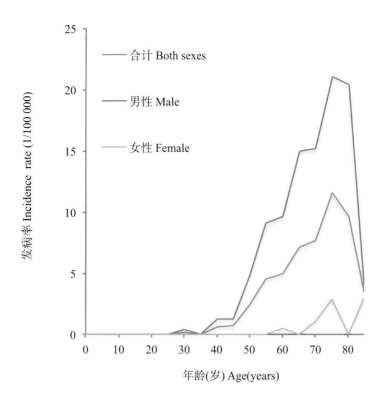

图 5.9.3 2017 年北京市郊区户籍居民喉癌年龄别发病率
Figure 5.9.3 Age-specific incidence rates of larynx cancer in peri-urban areas of Beijing, 2017

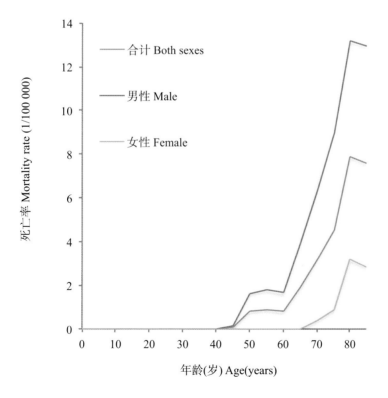

图 5.9.4 2017 年北京市户籍居民喉癌年龄别死亡率
Figure 5.9.4 Age-specific mortality rates of larynx cancer in Beijing, 2017

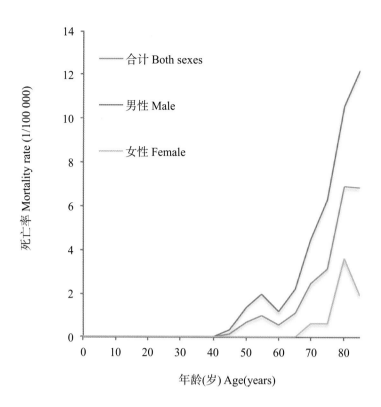

图 5.9.5 2017 年北京市城区户籍居民喉癌年龄别死亡率
Figure 5.9.5 Age-specific mortality rates of larynx cancer in urban areas of Beijing, 2017

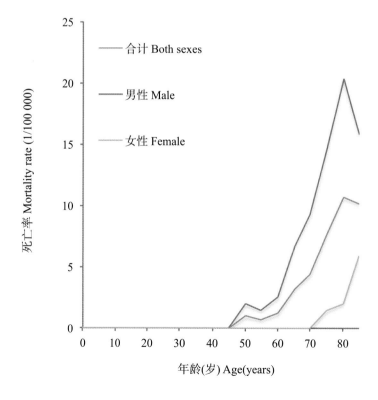

图 5.9.6 2017 年北京市郊区户籍居民喉癌年龄别死亡率
Figure 5.9.6 Age-specific mortality rates of larynx cancer in peri-urban areas of Beijing, 2017

（撰稿 李晴雨，校稿 张倩）

5.10 肺（C33-34）

2017年，北京市肺癌新发病例数为 10 125 例，占全部恶性肿瘤发病的 20.22%，位居恶性肿瘤发病第 2 位；其中男性 6 041 例，女性 4 084 例，城区 6 448 例，郊区 3 677 例。肺癌发病率为 74.39/10 万，中标发病率为 34.17/10 万，世标发病率为 33.94/10 万；男性世标发病率为女性的 1.54 倍，郊区世标发病率为城区的 1.07 倍。0~74 岁累积发病率为 4.12%（表 5.10.1）。

5.10 Lung (C33-34)

There were 10,125 new cases diagnosed as lung cancer (6,041 males and 4,084 females, 6,448 in urban areas and 3,677 in peri-urban areas), accounting for 20.22% of new cases of all cancers in 2017. Lung cancer was the 2nd common cancer in Beijing. The crude incidence rate was 74.39 per 100,000, with an ASR China and an ASR World of 34.17 and 33.94 per 100,000, respectively. The ASR World for incidence was 54% higher in males than in females and 7% higher in peri-urban areas than in urban area. The cumulative incidence rate for subjects aged 0 to 74 years was 4.12% (Table 5.10.1).

表 5.10.1 2017 年北京市户籍居民肺癌发病情况
Table 5.10.1 Incidence of lung cancer in Beijing, 2017

地区 Areas	性别 Sex	例数 No. cases	粗率 Crude rate （1/10^5）	构成比 Freq.（%）	中标率 ASR China （1/10^5）	世标率 ASR World （1/10^5）	累积率 Cumulative rate(0~74, %)	顺位 Rank
全市 All areas	合计 Both	10 125	74.39	20.22	34.17	33.94	4.12	2
	男性 Male	6 041	88.95	24.41	41.67	41.60	5.18	1
	女性 Female	4 084	59.89	16.13	27.38	26.95	3.13	2
城区 Urban areas	合计 Both	6 448	76.40	19.54	33.36	33.11	3.98	2
	男性 Male	3 718	88.32	23.07	38.98	38.91	4.79	1
	女性 Female	2 730	64.53	16.17	28.29	27.83	3.22	2
郊区 Peri-urban areas	合计 Both	3 677	71.12	21.54	35.82	35.58	4.34	1
	男性 Male	2 323	89.97	26.89	46.57	46.45	5.82	1
	女性 Female	1 354	52.31	16.05	25.99	25.63	2.99	2

2017 年，北京市肺癌死亡病例数为 7 390 例，占全部恶性肿瘤死亡的 28.37%，位居恶性肿瘤死亡第 1 位；其中男性 4 850 例，女性 2 540 例，城区 4 602 例，郊区 2 788 例。肺癌死亡率为 54.30/10 万，中标死亡率为 22.23/10 万，世标死亡率为 22.03/10 万；男性世标死亡率为女性的 2.23 倍，郊区世标死亡率为城区的 1.28 倍。0~74 岁累积死亡率为 2.49%（表 5.10.2）。

A total of 7,390 cases died of lung cancer (4,850 males and 2,540 females, 4,602 in urban areas and 2,788 in peri-urban areas), accounting for 28.37% of all cancer deaths in 2017, ranking the 1st among all cancers. The crude mortality rate was 54.30 per 100,000, with an ASR China rate and an ASR World rate of 22.23 and 22.03 per 100,000, respectively. The ASR World mortality was 123% higher in in males than in females and 28% higher in peri-urban areas than in urban areas, respectively. The cumulative mortality rate for subjects aged 0 to 74 years was 2.49% (Table 5.10.2).

表 5.10.2 2017 年北京市户籍居民肺癌死亡情况
Table 5.10.2 Mortality of lung cancer in Beijing, 2017

地区 Areas	性别 Sex	例数 No. deaths	粗率 Crude rate (1/10⁵)	构成比 Freq.（%）	中标率 ASR China (1/10⁵)	世标率 ASR World (1/10⁵)	累积率 Cumulative rate(0~74, %)	顺位 Rank
全市 All areas	合计 Both	7 390	54.30	28.37	22.23	22.03	2.49	1
	男性 Male	4 850	71.41	31.29	30.99	30.89	3.63	1
	女性 Female	2 540	37.25	24.08	14.16	13.84	1.42	1
城区 Urban areas	合计 Both	4 602	54.52	27.09	20.15	20.03	2.23	1
	男性 Male	3 013	71.57	30.18	28.03	28.08	3.25	1
	女性 Female	1 589	37.56	22.69	12.86	12.52	1.27	1
郊区 Peri-urban areas	合计 Both	2 788	53.93	30.77	25.98	25.63	2.91	1
	男性 Male	1 837	71.15	33.29	36.18	35.75	4.24	1
	女性 Female	951	36.74	26.84	16.59	16.31	1.68	1

北京市肺癌世标发病率由 2008 年的 32.26/10万上升到 2017 年的 33.94/10 万，10 年间发病率年均变化百分比仅为 0.18%，发病率变化趋势呈平台期，差异无统计学意义（P=0.495）；男性和女性 10 年间发病率年均变化百分比分别为 -0.38%（P=0.116）和 1.08%（P=0.013）。北京市肺癌世标死亡率由2008 年的 23.95/10 万下降到 2017 年的 22.03/10万，年均变化百分比为 -1.23%（P=0.006）；男性和女性 10 年间死亡率年均变化百分比分别为 -0.65%（P=0.055）和 -2.34%（P=0.001）。

肺癌年龄别发病率和死亡率在 40 岁以前均较低，40 岁以后快速上升，男性年龄别发病率上升速度高于女性（图 5.10.1 至图 5.10.6）。男性的肺癌发病率和死亡率均在 80~84 岁年龄组达到高峰，女性的肺癌发病率和死亡率均在 85 岁及以上年龄组达到高峰（图 5.10.1 和图 5.10.4）。城区和郊区年龄别发病率、死亡率变化有一定差别，但总体趋势相同（图 5.10.2 和图 5.10.3，图 5.10.5 和图 5.10.6）。

The ASR World for incidence of lung cancer increased from 32.26 per 100,000 in 2008 to 33.94 per 100,000 in 2017; the APC of ASR World for incidence was 0.18% (P=0.495) in the last decade. The APCs of ASR World for incidence of lung cancer in males and females were −0.38% (P=0.116) and 1.08% (P=0.013), respectively. The ASR World for mortality of lung cancer decreased from 23.95 per 100,000 in 2008 to 22.03 per 100,000 in 2017; the APC of ASR World for mortality was −1.23% (P=0.006). The APCs of ASR World for mortality of lung cancer in males and females were −0.65% (P=0.055) and −2.34% (P=0.001), respectively.

The age-specific incidence and mortality rates of lung cancer were relatively low at ages below 40 years, but at ages above 40 years, the rates increased sharply. The incidence rates grew faster in males than in females with the advancing of age (Figure 5.10.1-5.10.6). The age-specific incidence and mortality rates for males peaked at the age group of 80-84 years, and for females, the incidence and mortality rates peaked at the age group of 85 years and above (Figure 5.10.1, Figure 5.10.4). There were some differences in age-specific incidence and mortality rates between urban and peri-urban areas, but the overall trends were the same (Figure 5.10.2-5.10.3, Figure 5.10.5-5.10.6).

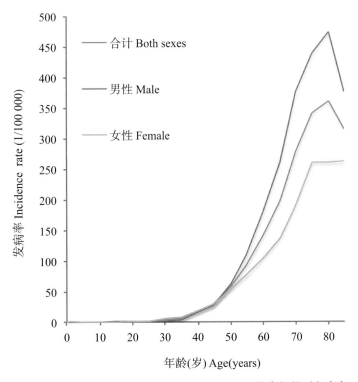

图 5.10.1 2017 年北京市户籍居民肺癌年龄别发病率
Figure 5.10.1 Age-specific incidence rates of lung cancer in Beijing, 2017

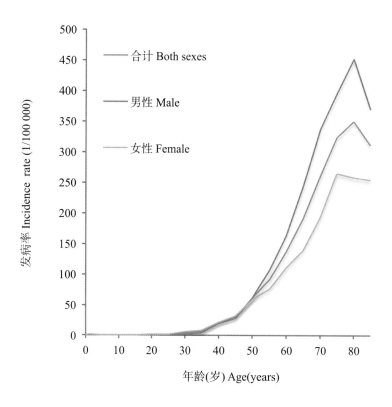

图 5.10.2 2017 年北京市城区户籍居民肺癌年龄别发病率

Figure 5.10.2 Age-specific incidence rates of lung cancer in urban areas of Beijing, 2017

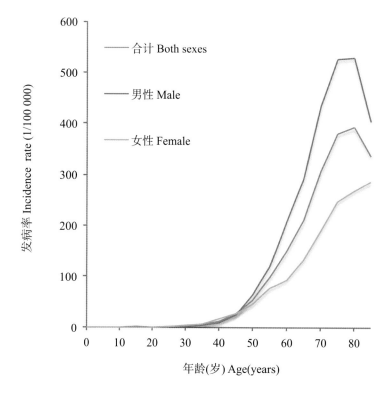

图 5.10.3 2017 年北京市郊区户籍居民肺癌年龄别发病率

Figure 5.10.3 Age-specific incidence rates of lung cancer in peri-urban areas of Beijing, 2017

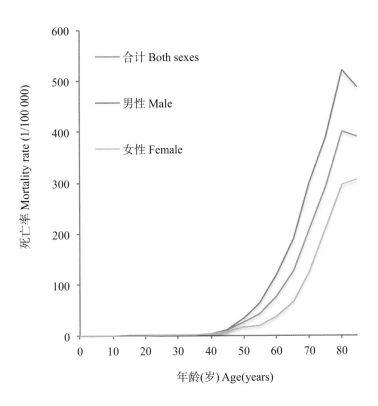

图 5.10.4 2017 年北京市户籍居民肺癌年龄别死亡率

Figure 5.10.4 Age-specific mortality rates of lung cancer in Beijing, 2017

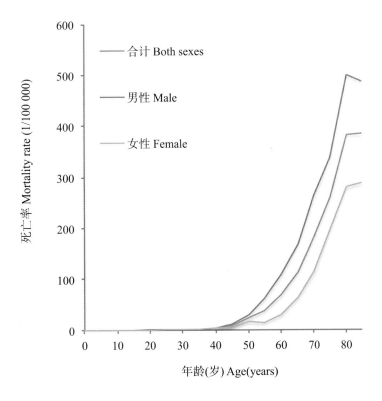

图 5.10.5 2017 年北京市城区户籍居民肺癌年龄别死亡率

Figure 5.10.5 Age-specific mortality rates of lung cancer in urban areas of Beijing, 2017

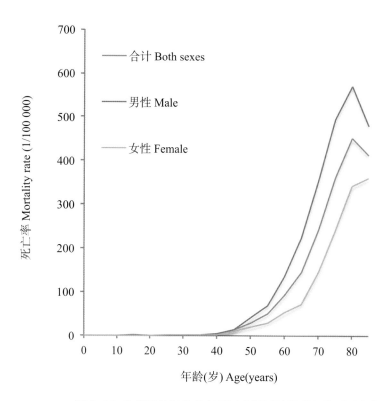

图 5.10.6　2017 年北京市郊区户籍居民肺癌年龄别死亡率

Figure 5.10.6 Age-specific mortality rates of lung cancer in peri-urban areas of Beijing, 2017

2017 年，北京市肺癌世标发病率和死亡率在 16 个辖区间有一定差异，郊区发病率和死亡率均高于城区（图 5.10.7 和图 5.10.8）。

In 2017, there were some differences between the 16 districts in ASR World for incidence and mortality of lung cancer in Beijing. Both the incidence and mortality rates were higher in peri-urban areas than in urban areas (Figure 5.10.7-5.10.8).

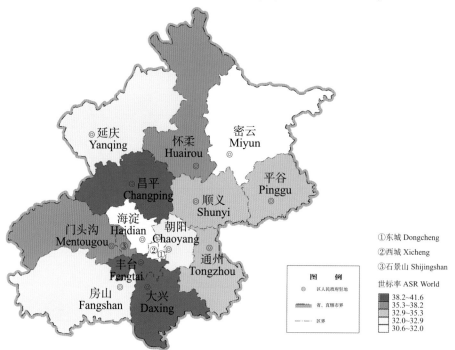

图 5.10.7　2017 年北京市户籍居民肺癌发病率（1/10⁵）地区分布情况

Figure 5.10.7 Incidence rates of lung cancer by district in Beijing, 2017 (1/10^5)

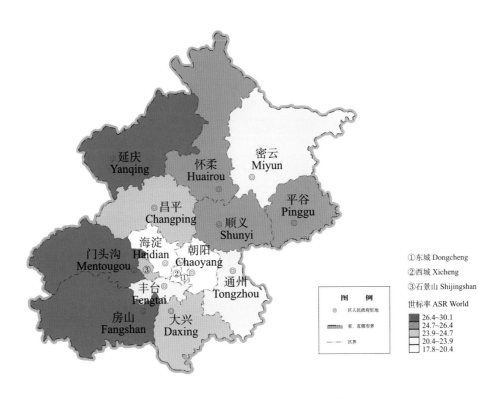

图 5.10.8 2017 年北京市户籍居民肺癌死亡率 (1/10^5) 地区分布情况
Figure 5.10.8 Mortality rates of lung cancer by district in Beijing, 2017 (1/10^5)

全部肺癌新发病例中，有明确亚部位的病例数占 50.11%。其中肺上叶是最常见的肺癌发病亚部位，占 54.79%；其后依次为下叶和中叶，分别占 35.85% 和 6.60%（图 5.10.9）。

About 50.11% cases were assigned to specified categories of lung cancer sites. Among those, upper lobe was the most common subsite, accounting for 54.79% of all cases, followed by the lower lobe (35.85%) and the middle lobe (6.60%) (Figure 5.10.9).

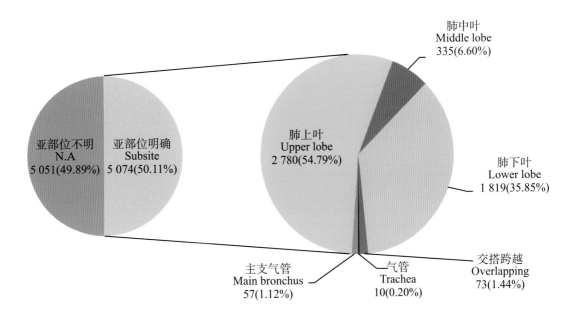

图 5.10.9 2017 年北京市户籍居民肺癌亚部位分布情况
Figure 5.10.9 Subsite distribution of lung cancer in Beijing, 2017

（撰稿 杨雷，校稿 程杨杨）

5.11 骨 (C40-41)

　　2017 年，北京市骨癌新发病例数为 164 例，占全部恶性肿瘤发病的 0.33%，位居恶性肿瘤发病第 21 位；其中男性 103 例，女性 61 例，城区 95 例，郊区 69 例。骨癌发病率为 1.20/10 万，中标发病率为 0.99/10 万，世标发病率为 0.95/10 万；男性世标发病率为女性的 2.15 倍，郊区世标发病率为城区的 1.43 倍。0~74 岁累积发病率为 0.08%（表 5.11.1）。

5.11 Bone (C40-41)

　　There were 164 new cases diagnosed as bone cancer (103 males and 61 females, 95 in urban areas and 69 in peri-urban areas), accounting for 0.33% of new cases of all cancers in 2017. Bone cancer was the 21st common cancer in Beijing. The crude incidence rate was 1.20 per 100,000, with an ASR China and an ASR World of 0.99 and 0.95 per 100,000, respectively. The ASR World for incidence was 115% higher in males than in females and 43% higher in peri-urban areas than in urban areas. The cumulative incidence rate for subjects aged 0 to 74 years was 0.08% (Table 5.11.1).

表 5.11.1 2017 年北京市户籍居民骨癌发病情况
Table 5.11.1 Incidence of bone cancer in Beijing, 2017

地区 Areas	性别 Sex	例数 No. cases	粗率 Crude rate （1/10⁵）	构成比 Freq.（%）	中标率 ASR China （1/10⁵）	世标率 ASR World （1/10⁵）	累积率 Cumulative rate(0~74, %)	顺位 Rank
全市 All areas	合计 Both	164	1.20	0.33	0.99	0.95	0.08	21
	男性 Male	103	1.52	0.42	1.34	1.29	0.10	17
	女性 Female	61	0.89	0.24	0.63	0.60	0.06	19
城区 Urban areas	合计 Both	95	1.13	0.29	0.88	0.82	0.07	21
	男性 Male	61	1.45	0.38	1.22	1.15	0.08	17
	女性 Female	34	0.80	0.20	0.52	0.48	0.05	20
郊区 Peri-urban areas	合计 Both	69	1.33	0.40	1.18	1.17	0.10	21
	男性 Male	42	1.63	0.49	1.55	1.53	0.13	17
	女性 Female	27	1.04	0.32	0.81	0.80	0.08	19

2017 年，北京市骨癌死亡病例数为 113 例，占全部恶性肿瘤死亡的 0.43%，位居恶性肿瘤死亡第 21 位；其中男性 64 例，女性 49 例，城区 50 例，郊区 63 例。骨癌死亡率为 0.83/10 万，中标死亡率为 0.51/10 万，世标死亡率为 0.49/10 万；男性世标死亡率为女性的 1.63 倍，郊区世标死亡率为城区的 1.84 倍。0~74 岁累积死亡率为 0.05%（表 5.11.2）。

A total of 113 cases died of bone cancer (64 males and 49 females, 50 in urban areas and 63 in peri-urban areas), accounting for 0.43% of all cancer deaths in 2017. Bone cancer was the 21st leading cause of cancer deaths in all cancers. The crude mortality rate was 0.83 per 100,000, with an ASR China and an ASR World of 0.51 and 0.49 per 100,000, respectively. The ASR World for mortality was 63% higher in males than in females and 84% higher in peri-urban areas than in urban areas. The cumulative mortality rate for subjects aged 0 to 74 years was 0.05% (Table 5.11.2).

表 5.11.2 2017 年北京市户籍居民骨癌死亡情况
Table 5.11.2 Mortality of bone cancer in Beijing, 2017

地区 Areas	性别 Sex	例数 No. deaths	粗率 Crude rate （1/10^5）	构成比 Freq.（%）	中标率 ASR China （1/10^5）	世标率 ASR World （1/10^5）	累积率 Cumulative rate(0~74, %)	顺位 Rank
全市 All areas	合计 Both	113	0.83	0.43	0.51	0.49	0.05	21
	男性 Male	64	0.94	0.41	0.62	0.60	0.05	18
	女性 Female	49	0.72	0.46	0.40	0.37	0.04	19
城区 Urban areas	合计 Both	50	0.59	0.29	0.41	0.38	0.03	23
	男性 Male	34	0.81	0.34	0.56	0.54	0.04	18
	女性 Female	16	0.38	0.23	0.26	0.22	0.02	21
郊区 Peri-urban areas	合计 Both	63	1.22	0.70	0.72	0.70	0.07	19
	男性 Male	30	1.16	0.54	0.77	0.75	0.07	16
	女性 Female	33	1.28	0.93	0.66	0.64	0.08	17

北京市骨癌 2008 年的世标发病率为 0.97/10 万，2017 年为 0.95/10 万，年均变化百分比为 3.03%（P=0.072）；男性和女性发病 10 年间年均变化百分比分别为 3.56%（P=0.076）和 1.93%

The incidence of ASR World of bone cancer was 0.97 per 100,000 in 2008 and 0.95 per 100,000 in 2017; the APC of ASR World for incidence was 3.03% (P=0.072). The APCs of ASR World for incidence of bone cancer in males and females were 3.56% (P=0.076) and 1.93% (P=0.399), respectively. The

（*P*=0.399）。北京市骨癌世标死亡率由 2008 年的 0.59/10 万下降到 2017 年的 0.49/10 万，年均变化百分比为 -1.93%（*P*=0.248）；男性和女性死亡 10 年间年均变化百分比分别为 -2.96%（*P*=0.077）和 -0.34%（*P*=0.902）。

　　骨癌年龄别发病率和死亡率均呈现"双峰"特征，15~19 岁组出现一个小高峰，在 55 岁之前处于较低水平，55 岁之后开始迅速上升，至 80~84 岁年龄组达到高峰，70 岁之后波动较大（图 5.11.1 至图 5.11.6）。整个年龄周期总体呈现男性骨癌发病率和死亡率高于女性（图 5.11.1 和图 5.11.4）。城区和郊区年龄别发病率、死亡率变化有一定差别，但总体趋势相同，城区波动较为明显（图 5.11.2 和图 5.11.3，图 5.11.5 和图 5.11.6）。

mortality of ASR World of bone cancer decreased from 0.59 per 100,000 in 2008 to 0.49 per 100,000 in 2017; the APC of ASR World for mortality was -1.93% (*P*=0.248). The APCs of ASR World for mortality of bone cancer in males and females were -2.96% (*P*=0.077) and -0.34% (*P*=0.902), respectively.

The age-specific incidence and mortality rates of bone cancer showed a double-peak phenomenon (Figure 5.11.1- 5.11.6). The first peak appeared at the age of 15-19 years old, after that the rates remained low in people below 55 years old, and the rates increased dramatically in people older than that. The rates reached the second peak at the age of 80-84 years old and showed big fluctuations after 70 years old. The incidence and mortality rates in males were higher than those in females across almost all age groups (Figure 5.11.1, Figure 5.11.4). There were some differences in age-specific incidence and mortality rates between urban and peri-urban areas, but the overall trends were same. The age-specific incidence and mortality rates in urban areas showed huge fluctuations (Figure 5.11.2-5.11.3, Figure 5.11.5-5.11.6).

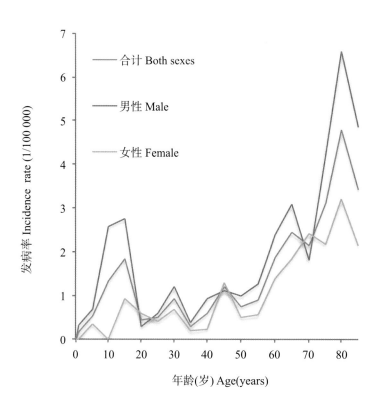

图 5.11.1 2017 年北京市户籍居民骨癌年龄别发病率
Figure 5.11.1 Age-specific incidence rates of bone cancer in Beijing, 2017

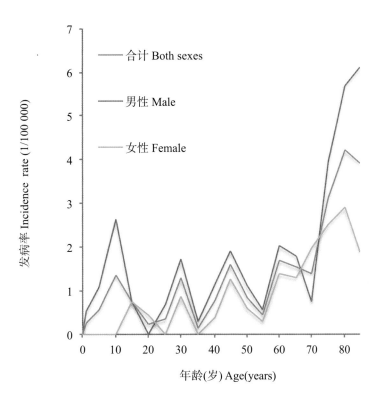

图 5.11.2 2017 年北京市城区户籍居民骨癌年龄别发病率
Figure 5.11.2 Age-specific incidence rates of bone cancer in urban areas of Beijing, 2017

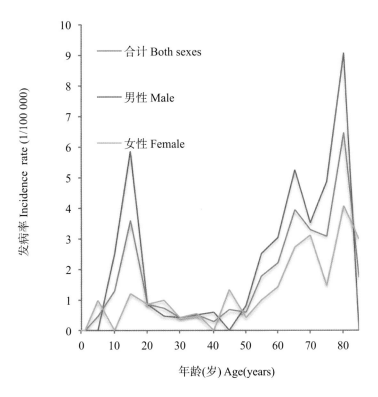

图 5.11.3 2017 年北京市郊区户籍居民骨癌年龄别发病率
Figure 5.11.3 Age-specific incidence rates of bone cancer in peri-urban areas of Beijing, 2017

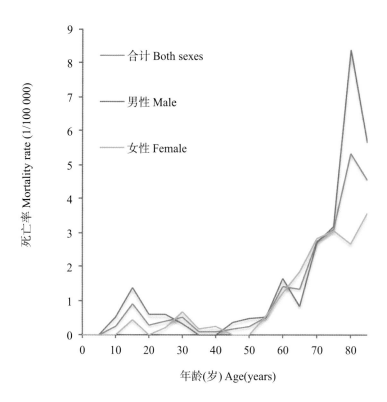

图 5.11.4 2017 年北京市户籍居民骨癌年龄别死亡率
Figure 5.11.4 Age-specific mortality rates of bone cancer in Beijing, 2017

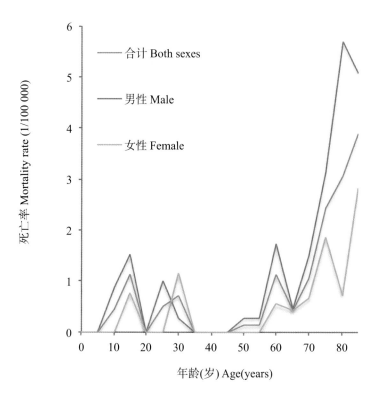

图 5.11.5 2017 年北京市城区户籍居民骨癌年龄别死亡率
Figure 5.11.5 Age-specific mortality rates of bone cancer in urban areas of Beijing, 2017

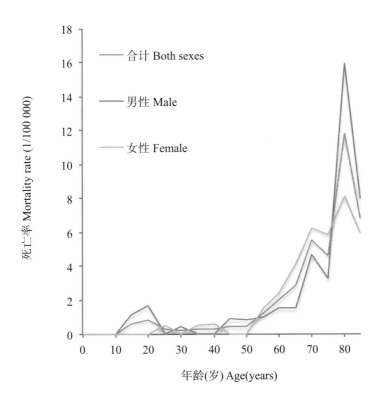

图 5.11.6　2017 年北京市郊区户籍居民骨癌年龄别死亡率
Figure 5.11.6 Age-specific mortality rates of bone cancer in peri-urban areas of Beijing, 2017

全部骨癌新发病例中，28.66% 的骨癌发生在四肢的骨和关节软骨，71.34% 发生在其他和未特指部位的骨和关节软骨（图 5.11.7）。

For subsites, about 28.66% of bone cancer occurred in bone and articular cartilage of limbs, and 71.34% bone cancer developed in other and unspecified sites (Figure 5.11.7).

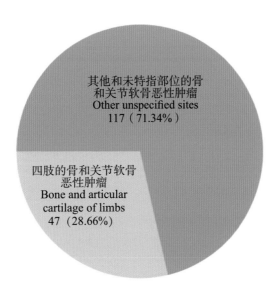

图 5.11.7　2017 年北京市户籍居民骨癌亚部位分布情况
Figure 5.11.7 Subsite distribution of bone cancer in Beijing, 2017

（撰稿　李晴雨，校稿　张倩）

5.12 女性乳腺 (C50)

　　2017 年，北京市女性乳腺癌新发病例数为 5 119 例，占女性全部恶性肿瘤发病的 20.22%，位居女性恶性肿瘤发病第 1 位；其中城区 3 468 例，郊区 1 651 例。女性乳腺癌发病率为 75.07/10 万，中标发病率为 46.27/10 万，世标发病率为 43.45/10 万；城区世标发病率为郊区的 1.22 倍。0~74 岁累积发病率为 4.79%（表 5.12.1）。

5.12 Female Breast (C50)

There were 5,119 new cases diagnosed as female breast cancer (3,468 in urban areas and 1,651 in peri-urban areas), accounting for 20.22% of new cases of all cancers among females in 2017. Breast cancer was the most common cancer among females in Beijing. The crude incidence rate was 75.07 per 100,000, with an ASR China and an ASR World of 46.27 and 43.45 per 100,000, respectively. The ASR World for incidence was 22% higher in urban areas than that in peri-urban areas. The cumulative incidence rate for subjects aged 0 to 74 years was 4.79% (Table 5.12.1).

表 5.12.1 2017 年北京市户籍居民女性乳腺癌发病情况
Table 5.12.1 Incidence of female breast cancer in Beijing, 2017

地区 Areas	例数 No. cases	粗率 Crude rate $(1/10^5)$	构成比 Freq.（%）	中标率 ASR China $(1/10^5)$	世标率 ASR World $(1/10^5)$	累积率 Cumulative rate(0~74, %)	顺位 Rank
全市 All areas	5 119	75.07	20.22	46.27	43.45	4.79	1
城区 Urban areas	3 468	81.97	20.54	49.50	46.65	5.20	1
郊区 Peri-urban areas	1 651	63.79	19.58	40.89	38.10	4.14	1

　　2017 年，北京市女性乳腺癌死亡病例数为 1 067 例，占女性全部恶性肿瘤死亡的 10.12%，位居女性恶性肿瘤死亡第 3 位；其中城区 745 例，郊区 322 例。女性乳腺癌死亡率为 15.65/10 万，中标死亡率为 7.40/10 万，世标死亡率为 7.29/10 万；城区世标死亡率为郊区的 1.22 倍。0~74 岁累积死亡率为 0.81%（表 5.12.2）。

A total of 1,067 female cases died of breast cancer (745 in urban areas and 322 in peri-urban areas), accounting for 10.12% of all cancer deaths among females in 2017. Female breast cancer was the 3rd leading cause of cancer deaths in all cancers among females. The crude mortality rate was 15.65 per 100,000, with an ASR China and an ASR World of 7.40 and 7.29 per 100,000, respectively. The ASR World for mortality in urban areas was 22% higher than that in peri-urban areas. The cumulative mortality rate for subjects aged 0 to 74 years was 0.81% (Table 5.12.2).

表 5.12.2 2017 年北京市户籍居民女性乳腺癌死亡情况
Table 5.12.2 Mortality of female breast cancer in Beijing, 2017

地区 Areas	例数 No. deaths	粗率 Crude rate (1/10⁵)	构成比 Freq.（%）	中标率 ASR China (1/10⁵)	世标率 ASR World (1/10⁵)	累积率 Cumulative rate(0~74, %)	顺位 Rank
全市 All areas	1 067	15.65	10.12	7.40	7.29	0.81	3
城区 Urban areas	745	17.61	10.64	7.90	7.82	0.90	3
郊区 Peri-urban areas	322	12.44	9.09	6.59	6.39	0.68	3

北京市女性乳腺癌世标发病率由 2008 年的 36.18/10 万上升到 2017 年的 43.45/10 万，年均变化百分比为 2.03%（P<0.001）；女性乳腺癌世标死亡率由 2008 年的 6.33/10 万上升到 2017 年的 7.29/10 万，年均变化百分比为 1.32%（P=0.003）。

女性乳腺癌发病率自 20~24 岁组开始快速升高，城区和郊区虽均在 60~64 岁组达到高峰，但城区和郊区年龄别发病率呈现不同的特点：城区 65~74 岁组年龄别发病率仍处于较高水平，后逐渐下降；但郊区呈现明显的"双峰分布"，年龄别发病率在 65~69 岁组有所下降后，于 70~74 岁组上升形成第二个高峰，自74~79岁组开始逐渐下降（图 5.12.1 至图 5.12.3）。女性乳腺癌年龄别死亡率自 25~29 岁组开始快速上升，城区和郊区虽然在高年龄组略有波动，但整体年龄别死亡率呈现递增趋势，均在 85 岁及以上年龄组达到高峰（图5.12.4 至图 5.12.6）。

The ASR World for incidence of female breast cancer increased from 36.18 per 100,000 in 2008 to 43.45 per 100,000 in 2017. The APC of ASR World for incidence was 2.03% (P<0.001). The ASR World for mortality of female breast cancer increased from 6.33 per 100,000 in 2008 to 7.29 per 100,000 in 2017. The APC of ASR World for mortality was 1.32% (P=0.003).

The age-specific incidence rate of female breast cancer increased dramatically for age groups above 24 years and peaked at the age group of 60-64 years in urban and peri-urban areas. However, the age-specific incidence rates for female breast cancer in urban and peri-urban areas showed different characteristics: in urban areas, the age-specific incidence rate was still high at the age group of 65-74 years but decreased in age groups above 75 years; and in the peri-urban areas, the age-specific incidence rates showed a double-peak pattern, where the age-specific incidence rate at the age group of 70~74 years peaked again after it declined somewhat at the age group of 65~69 years, and decreased at the age groups above 74 years (Figure 5.12.1-5.12.3). The age-specific mortality rate of female breast cancer increased sharply in the age groups of 25 years and above. Though there was some fluctuation in the older age groups, the age-specific mortality rate increased with the advancing of age in general and peaked at the 85+ age group in urban and peri-urban areas (Figure 5.12.4-5.12.6).

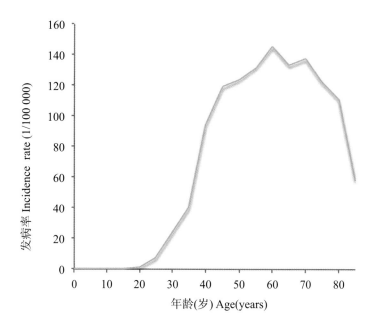

图 5.12.1 2017 年北京市户籍居民女性乳腺癌年龄别发病率
Figure 5.12.1 Age-specific incidence rate of female breast cancer in Beijing, 2017

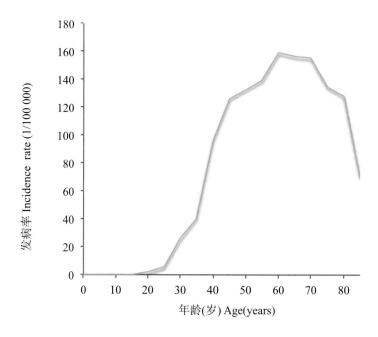

图 5.12.2 2017 年北京市城区户籍居民女性乳腺癌年龄别发病率
Figure 5.12.2 Age-specific incidence rate of female breast cancer in urban areas of Beijing, 2017

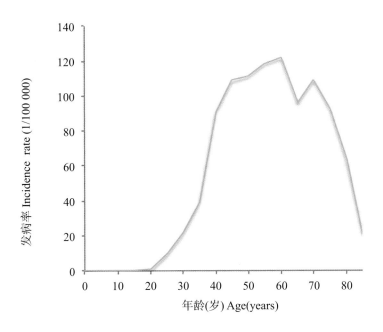

图 5.12.3 2017 年北京市郊区户籍居民女性乳腺癌年龄别发病率
Figure 5.12.3 Age-specific incidence rate of female breast cancer in peri-urban areas of Beijing, 2017

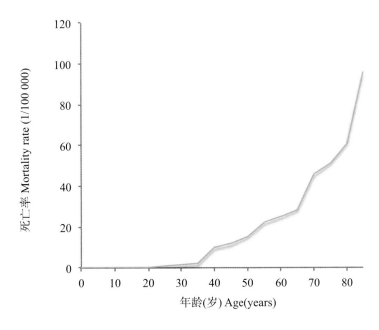

图 5.12.4 2017 年北京市户籍居民女性乳腺癌年龄别死亡率
Figure 5.12.4 Age-specific mortality rate of female breast cancer in Beijing, 2017

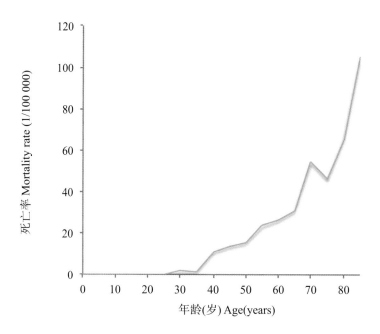

图 5.12.5 2017 年北京市城区户籍居民女性乳腺癌年龄别死亡率

Figure 5.12.5 Age-specific mortality rate of female breast cancer in urban areas of Beijing, 2017

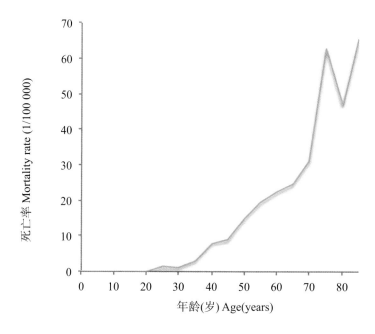

图 5.12.6 2017 年北京市郊区户籍居民女性乳腺癌年龄别死亡率

Figure 5.12.6 Age-specific mortality rate of female breast cancer in peri-urban areas of Beijing, 2017

2017 年，北京市女性乳腺癌世标发病率和死亡率在 16 个辖区间有显著差异，城区发病率和死亡率均高于郊区（图 5.12.7 和图 5.12.8）。

In 2017, there were significant differences between the 16 districts in ASR World for incidence and mortality of female breast cancer in Beijing. The incidence and mortality rates were higher in urban areas than in peri-urban areas (Figure 5.12.7–5.12.8).

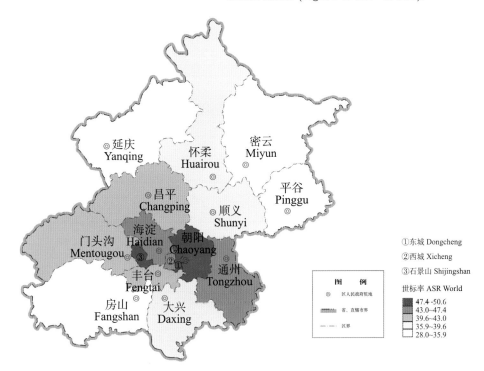

图 5.12.7 2017 年北京市户籍居民女性乳腺癌发病率（1/10⁵）地区分布情况
Figure 5.12.7 Incidence rates of female breast cancer by district in Beijing, 2017（1/10⁵）

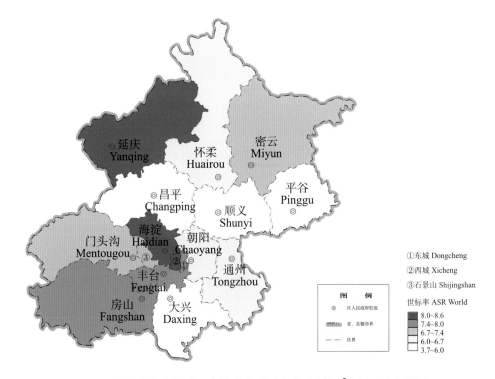

图 5.12.8 2017 年北京市户籍居民女性乳腺癌死亡率（1/10⁵）地区分布情况
Figure 5.12.8 Mortality rates of female breast cancer by district in Beijing, 2017（1/10⁵）

全部女性乳腺癌新发病例中，有明确亚部位的病例数占 59.37%。其中乳腺上外象限是最常见的发病部位，占 48.63%；其后依次为上内象限（18.20%）、交搭跨越（11.62%）、下外象限（11.58%）、下内象限（6.68%）、中央部（2.04%）以及乳头和乳晕（1.25%）（图 5.12.9）。

About 59.37% cases were assigned to specified categories of female breast cancer sites. Among those, upper outer quadrant of breast was the most common site, accounting for 48.63% of all cases, followed by the upper inner (18.20%), the overlapping (11.62%), the lower outer (11.58%), the lower inner (6.68%), the central portion (2.04%) and the nipple and areola (1.25%) (Figure 5.12.9).

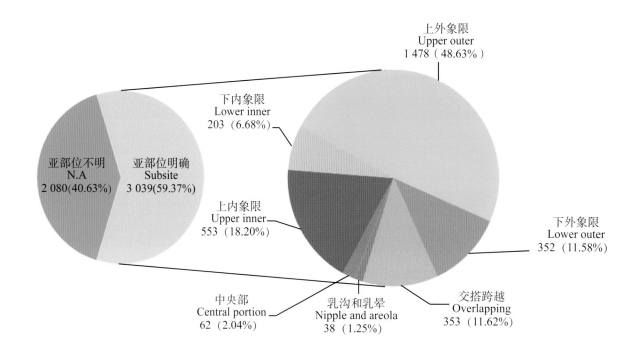

图 5.12.9 2017 年北京市户籍居民女性乳腺癌亚部位分布情况
Figure 5.12.9 Subsite distribution of female breast cancer in Beijing, 2017

（撰稿 刘硕，校稿 李慧超）

5.13 子宫颈 (C53)

2017 年，北京市子宫颈癌新发病例数为 652 例，占女性全部恶性肿瘤发病的 2.58%，位居女性恶性肿瘤发病第 10 位；其中城区 391 例，郊区 261 例。子宫颈癌发病率为 9.56/10 万，中标发病率为 6.92/10 万，世标发病率为 6.17/10 万；郊区世标发病率为城区的 1.11 倍。0~74 岁累积发病率为 0.61%（表 5.13.1）。

5.13 Cervix (C53)

There were 652 new cases diagnosed as cervical cancer (391 in urban areas and 261 in peri-urban areas), accounting for 2.58% of new female cases of all cancers in 2017. Cervical cancer was the 10th common female cancer in Beijing. The crude incidence rate was 9.56 per 100,000, with an ASR China and an ASR World of 6.92 and 6.17 per 100,000, respectively. The ASR world for incidence was 11% higher in peri-urban areas than in urban areas. The cumulative incidence rate for subjects aged 0 to 74 years was 0.61% (Table 5.13.1).

表 5.13.1　2017 年北京市户籍居民子宫颈癌发病情况
Table 5.13.1 Incidence of cervical cancer in Beijing, 2017

地区 Areas	例数 No. cases	粗率 Crude rate (1/10^5)	构成比 Freq. (%)	中标率 ASR China (1/10^5)	世标率 ASR World (1/10^5)	累积率 Cumulative rate(0~74, %)	顺位 Rank
全市 All areas	652	9.56	2.58	6.92	6.17	0.61	10
城区 Urban areas	391	9.24	2.32	6.58	5.92	0.59	12
郊区 Peri-urban areas	261	10.08	3.09	7.51	6.59	0.64	8

2017 年，北京市子宫颈癌死亡病例数为 237 例，占女性全部恶性肿瘤死亡的 2.25%，位居女性恶性肿瘤死亡第 14 位；其中城区 140 例，郊区 97 例。子宫颈癌死亡率为 3.48/10 万，中标死亡率为 2.07/10 万，世标死亡率为 1.92/10 万；郊区世标死亡率为城区的 1.20 倍。0~74 岁累积死亡率为 0.20%（表 5.13.2）。

A total of 237 cases died of cervical cancer (140 in urban areas and 97 in peri-urban areas), accounting for 2.25% of all female cancer deaths in 2017. Cervical cancer was the 14th leading cause of cancer deaths in all female cancers. The crude mortality rate was 3.48 per 100,000, with an ASR China and an ASR World of 2.07 and 1.92 per 100,000, respectively. The ASR World for mortality was 20% higher in peri-urban areas than in urban areas. The cumulative mortality rate for subjects aged 0 to 74 years was 0.20% (Table 5.13.2).

表 5.13.2 2017 年北京市户籍居民子宫颈癌死亡情况
Table 5.13.2 Mortality of cervical cancer in Beijing, 2017

地区 Areas	例数 No. deaths	粗率 Crude rate (1/10⁵)	构成比 Freq. (%)	中标率 ASR China (1/10⁵)	世标率 ASR World (1/10⁵)	累积率 Cumulative rate(0~74, %)	顺位 Rank
全市 All areas	237	3.48	2.25	2.07	1.92	0.20	14
城区 Urban areas	140	3.31	2.00	1.94	1.78	0.18	14
郊区 Peri-urban areas	97	3.75	2.74	2.29	2.14	0.22	11

北京市子宫颈癌世标发病率由 2008 年的 5.22/10 万上升到 2017 年的 6.17/10 万，年均变化百分比为 2.24%（P=0.011）。北京市子宫颈癌世标死亡率由 2008 年的 1.35/10 万上升到 2017 年的 1.92/10 万，年均变化百分比为 3.82%（P=0.002）。

子宫颈癌年龄别发病率在 20 岁以前处于较低水平，20 岁以后快速上升，至 50~54 岁年龄组达高峰，之后逐渐下降（图 5.13.1）。年龄别死亡率在 20 岁以前处于较低水平，20 岁以后随年龄的增加逐渐升高，在 50~54 岁年龄组出现一个小高峰，随后降低，60 岁之后再次迅速上升，至 80~84 岁年龄组达到高峰（图 5.13.4）。城区和郊区年龄别发病率、死亡率变化有一定差别，但总体趋势相同，郊区波动较为明显（图 5.13.2 和图 5.13.3，图 5.13.5 和图 5.13.6）。

The incidence of ASR World of cervical cancer increased from 5.22 per 100,000 in 2008 to 6.17 per 100,000 in 2017; the APC of ASR World for incidence was 2.24% (P=0.011). The mortality of ASR World of cervical cancer increased from 1.35 per 100,000 in 2008 to 1.92 per 100,000 in 2017; the APC of ASR World for mortality was 3.82% (P=0.002).

The age-specific incidence rates of cervical cancer were relatively low in people below 20 years old, and the rate increased sharply in people older than that (Figure 5.13.1). It reached peak at the age group of 50-54 years, and then decreased gradually. The age-specific mortality rates of cervical cancer were low in people below 20 years old and gradually increased with age. The first peak appeared at the age group of 50-54 years old, after that the rate decreased before 60 years old. But it increased dramatically since then, reaching the second peak at the age group of 80-84 years (Figure 5.13.4). There were some differences in age-specific incidence and mortality rates between urban and peri-urban areas, but the overall trends were same. The age-specific incidence and mortality rates in peri-urban areas showed huge fluctuations (Figure 5.13.2-5.13.3, Figure 5.13.5-5.13.6).

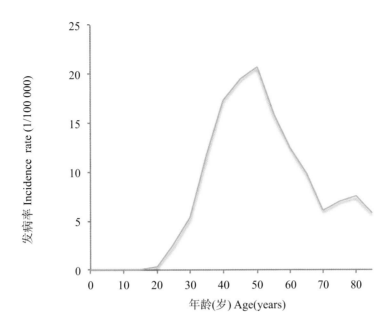

图 5.13.1 2017 年北京市户籍居民子宫颈癌年龄别发病率
Figure 5.13.1 Age-specific incidence rate of cervical cancer in Beijing, 2017

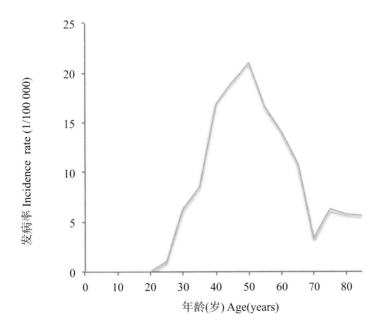

图 5.13.2 2017 年北京市城区户籍居民子宫颈癌年龄别发病率
Figure 5.13.2 Age-specific incidence rate of cervical cancer in urban areas of Beijing, 2017

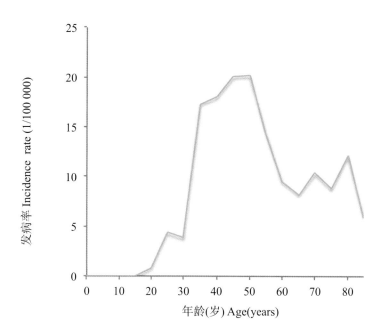

图 5.13.3 2017 年北京市郊区户籍居民子宫颈癌年龄别发病率
Figure 5.13.3 Age-specific incidence rate of cervical cancer in peri-urban areas of Beijing, 2017

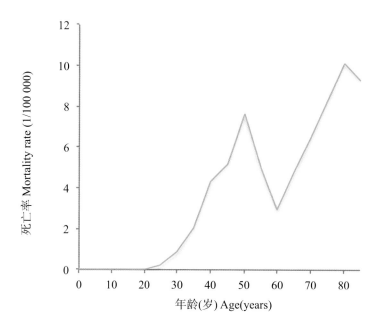

图 5.13.4 2017 年北京市户籍居民子宫颈癌年龄别死亡率
Figure 5.13.4 Age-specific mortality rate of cervical cancer in Beijing, 2017

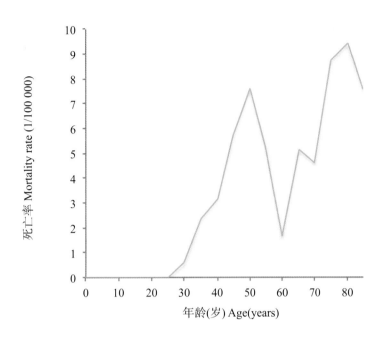

图 5.13.5 2017 年北京市城区户籍居民子宫颈癌年龄别死亡率
Figure 5.13.5 Age-specific mortality rate of cervical cancer in urban areas of Beijing, 2017

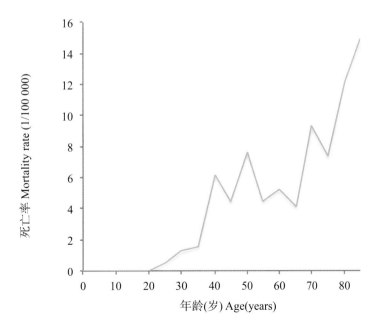

图 5.13.6 2017 年北京市郊区户籍居民子宫颈癌年龄别死亡率
Figure 5.13.6 Age-specific mortality rate of cervical cancer in peri-urban areas of Beijing, 2017

2017 年，北京市子宫颈癌世标发病率和死亡率在 16 个辖区间存在一定差异，郊区发病率和死亡率均高于城区（图 5.13.7 和图 5.13.8）。

In 2017, there were some differences between the 16 districts in ASR World for incidence and mortality of cervical cancer in Beijing. The incidence and mortality rates were higher in peri-urban areas than in urban areas (Figure 5.13.7–5.13.8).

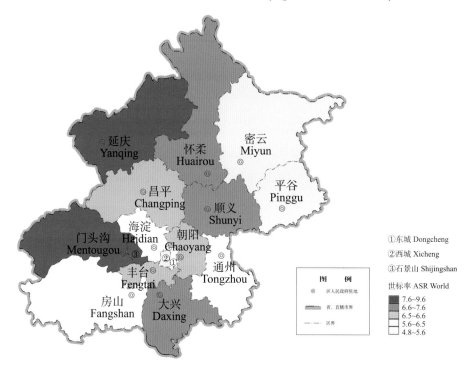

图 5.13.7 2017 年北京市户籍居民子宫颈癌发病率（1/10^5）地区分布情况

Figure 5.13.7 Incidence rates of cervical cancer by district in Beijing, 2017 (1/10^5)

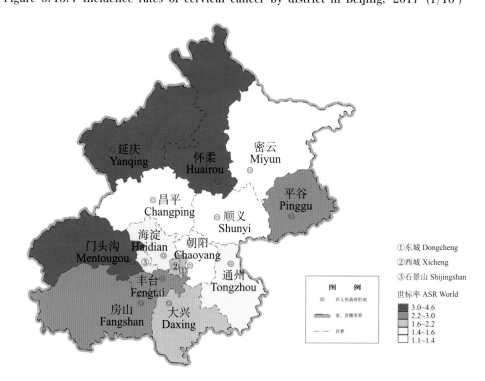

图 5.13.8 2017 年北京市户籍居民子宫颈癌死亡率（1/10^5）地区分布情况

Figure 5.13.8 Mortality rates of cervical cancer by district in Beijing, 2017 (1/10^5)

（撰稿 张希，校稿 李晴雨）

5.14 子宫体（C54-55）

5.14 Uterus (C54-55)

2017年，北京市子宫体癌新发病例数为1 358例，占女性全部恶性肿瘤发病的5.36%，位居女性恶性肿瘤发病第5位；其中城区853例，郊区505例。子宫体癌发病率为19.92/10万，中标发病率为11.77/10万，世标发病率为11.43/10万；城区世标发病率为郊区的1.01倍。0~74岁累积发病率为1.31%（表5.14.1）。

There were 1,358 new cases diagnosed as uterus cancer (853 in urban areas and 505 in peri-urban areas), accounting for 5.36% of new cases of all female cancers in 2017. Uterus cancer was the 5th common female cancer in Beijing. The crude incidence rate was 19.92 per 100,000, with an ASR China and an ASR World of 11.77 and 11.43 per 100,000, respectively. The ASR World for incidence was 1% higher in urban areas than in peri-urban areas. The cumulative incidence rate for subjects aged 0 to 74 years was 1.31% (Table 5.14.1).

表 5.14.1 2017 年北京市户籍居民子宫体癌发病情况
Table 5.14.1 Incidence of uterus cancer in Beijing, 2017

地区 Areas	例数 No. cases	粗率 Crude rate （1/10^5）	构成比 Freq.（%）	中标率 ASR China （1/10^5）	世标率 ASR World （1/10^5）	累积率 Cumulative rate(0~74, %）	顺位 Rank
全市 All areas	1 358	19.92	5.36	11.77	11.43	1.31	5
城区 Urban areas	853	20.16	5.05	11.73	11.44	1.34	5
郊区 Peri-urban areas	505	19.51	5.99	11.75	11.35	1.26	5

2017 年，北京市子宫体癌死亡病例数为240例，占女性全部恶性肿瘤死亡的2.28%，位居女性恶性肿瘤死亡第13位；其中城区170例，郊区70例。子宫体癌死亡率为3.52/10万，中标死亡率为1.61/10万，世标死亡率为1.59/10万；城区世标死亡率为郊区的1.26倍。0~74岁累积死亡率为0.20%（表5.14.2）。

A total of 240 cases died of uterus cancer (170 in urban areas and 70 in peri-urban areas), accounting for 2.28% of all female cancer deaths in 2017. Uterus cancer was the 13th leading cause of cancer deaths in all kinds of female cancers. The crude mortality rate was 3.52 per 100,000, with an ASR China and an ASR World of 1.61 and 1.59 per 100,000 respectively. The ASR World for mortality in urban areas were 26% higher than that in peri-urban areas. The cumulative mortality rate for subjects aged 0 to 74 years was 0.20% (Table 5.14.2).

表 5.14.2 2017 年北京市户籍居民子宫体癌死亡情况
Table 5.14.2 Mortality of uterus cancer in Beijing, 2017

地区 Areas	例数 No. deaths	粗率 Crude rate (1/10⁵)	构成比 Freq.（%）	中标率 ASR China (1/10⁵)	世标率 ASR World (1/10⁵)	累积率 Cumulative rate(0~74,%)	顺位 Rank
全市 All areas	240	3.52	2.28	1.61	1.59	0.20	13
城区 Urban areas	170	4.02	2.43	1.73	1.71	0.21	12
郊区 Peri-urban areas	70	2.70	1.98	1.38	1.36	0.18	15

北京市子宫体癌世标发病率由 2008 年的 7.83/10 万上升到 2017 年的 11.43/10 万，10 年间发病率年均变化百分比为 4.22%（*P*<0.001）。北京市子宫体癌世标死亡率由 2008 年的 1.38/10 万上升到 2017 年的 1.59/10 万，10 年间死亡率年均变化百分比为 0.22%（*P*=0.828）。

子宫体癌年龄别发病率在 25 岁以前处于较低水平，自 25 岁开始逐渐上升，35 岁以后快速上升，至 55~60 岁年龄组达高峰，之后逐渐下降（图 5.14.1）。年龄别死亡率在 40 岁以前处于较低水平，40 岁以后随年龄的增加逐渐升高，在 80~84 岁年龄组达到高峰（图 5.14.4）。城区和郊区年龄别发病率、死亡率变化有一定差别，但总体趋势相同，郊区波动较为明显（图 5.14.2 和图 5.14.3，图 5.14.5 和图 5.14.6）。

The ASR World for incidence of uterus cancer increased from 7.83 per 100,000 in 2008 to 11.43 per 100,000 in 2017; and the APC of ASR World for incidence was 4.22% (*P*<0.001). The ASR World for mortality of uterus cancer increased from 1.38 per 100,000 in 2008 to 1.59 per 100,000 in 2017; and the APC of ASR World for mortality was 0.22% (*P*=0.828).

The age-specific incidence rate of uterus cancer was relatively low before the age of 25 years, thereafter increased gradually and went up rapidly in people aged 35 years and above, peaking at the age group of 55-60 years with a gradual decline thereafter (Figure 5.14.1). The age-specific mortality rate of uterus cancer was low before 40 years old and gradually increased with advancing of age, peaking at the age group of 80-84 (Figure 5.14.4). There were some differences in age-specific incidence and mortality rates between urban and peri-urban areas, but the overall trends were same. The distribution of age-specific incidence and mortality rates in peri-urban areas showed huge fluctuations (Figure 5.14.2-5.14.3, Figure 5.14.5-5.14.6).

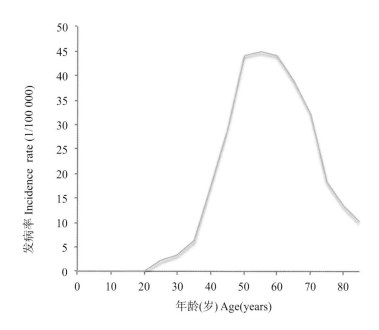

图 5.14.1 2017 年北京市户籍居民子宫体癌年龄别发病率
Figure 5.14.1 Age-specific incidence rate of uterus cancer in Beijing, 2017

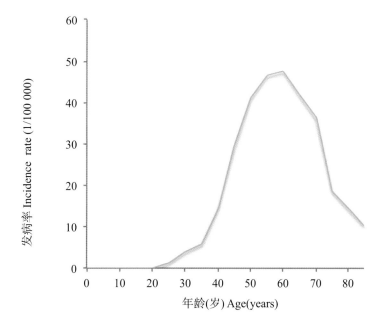

图 5.14.2 2017 年北京市城区户籍居民子宫体癌年龄别发病率
Figure 5.14.2 Age-specific incidence rate of uterus cancer in urban areas of Beijing, 2017

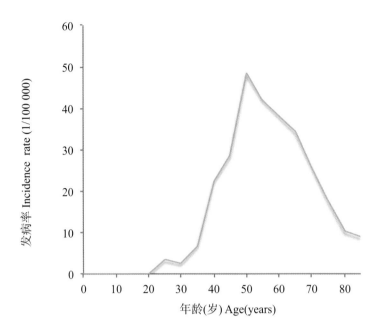

图 5.14.3 2017 年北京市郊区户籍居民子宫体癌年龄别发病率
Figure 5.14.3 Age-specific incidence rate of uterus cancer in peri-urban areas of Beijing, 2017

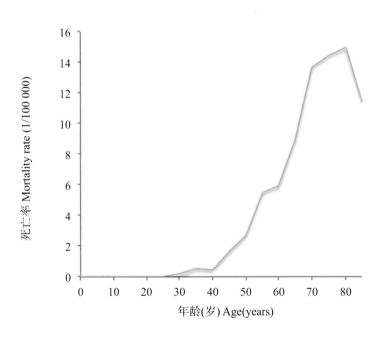

图 5.14.4 2017 年北京市户籍居民子宫体癌年龄别死亡率
Figure 5.14.4 Age-specific mortality rate of uterus cancer in Beijing, 2017

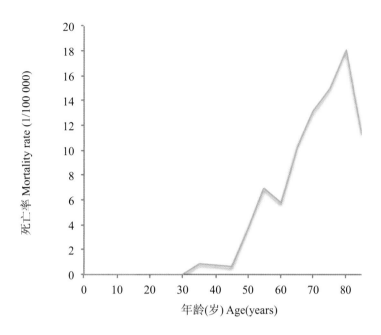

图 5.14.5 2017 年北京市城区户籍居民子宫体癌年龄别死亡率
Figure 5.14.5 Age-specific mortality rate of uterus cancer in urban areas of Beijing, 2017

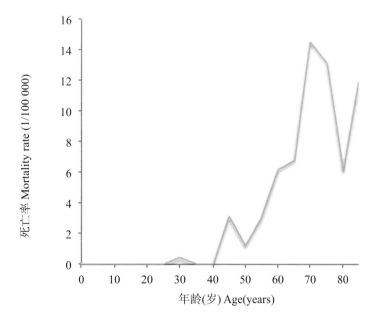

图 5.14.6 2017 年北京市郊区户籍居民子宫体癌年龄别死亡率
Figure 5.14.6 Age-specific mortality rate of uterus cancer in peri-urban areas of Beijing, 2017

2017 年，北京市子宫体癌世标发病率和死亡率在 16 个辖区间有一定差异，城区发病率和死亡率均高于郊区（图 5.14.7 和图 5.14.8）。

In 2017, there were some differences between the 16 districts in ASR World for incidence and mortality of uterus cancer in Beijing. The incidence and mortality rates of uterus cancer were higher in urban areas than in peri-urban areas (Figure 5.14.7-5.14.8).

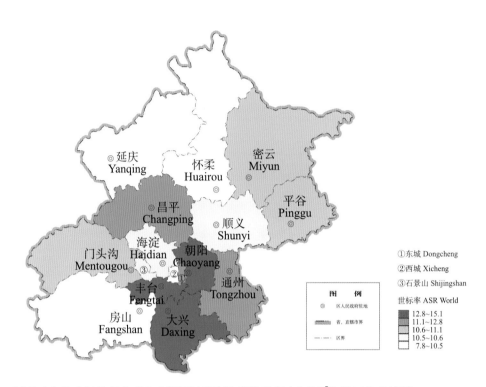

图 5.14.7 2017 年北京市户籍居民子宫体癌发病率（1/10⁵）地区分布情况
Figure 5.14.7 Incidence rates of uterus cancer by district in Beijing, 2017 (1/10^5)

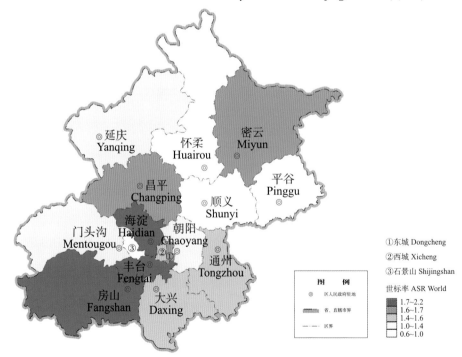

图 5.14.8 2017 年北京市户籍居民子宫体癌死亡率 (1/10⁵) 地区分布情况
Figure 5.14.8 Mortality rates of uterus cancer by district in Beijing, 2017 (1/10^5)

（撰稿 张希，校稿 程杨杨）

5.15 卵巢（C56）

2017 年，北京市卵巢癌新发病例数为 842 例，占女性全部恶性肿瘤发病的 3.33%，位居女性恶性肿瘤发病第 6 位；其中城区 544 例，郊区 298 例。卵巢癌发病率为 12.35/10 万，中标发病率为 7.57/10 万，世标发病率为 7.26/10 万；城区世标发病率为郊区的 1.09 倍。0~74 岁累积发病率为 0.79%（表 5.15.1）。

5.15 Ovary (C56)

There were 842 new cases diagnosed as ovarian cancer (544 in urban areas and 298 in peri-urban areas), accounting for 3.33% of new cases of all female cancers in 2017. Ovarian cancer was the 6th common female cancer in Beijing. The crude incidence rate was 12.35 per 100,000, with an ASR China and an ASR World of 7.57 and 7.26 per 100,000 respectively. The ASR World for incidence was 9% higher in urban areas than that in peri-urban areas. The cumulative incidence rate for subjects aged 0 to 74 years was 0.79% (Table 5.15.1).

表 5.15.1 2017 年北京市户籍居民卵巢癌发病情况
Table 5.15.1 Incidence of ovarian cancer in Beijing, 2017

地区 Areas	例数 No. cases	粗率 Crude rate (1/10^5)	构成比 Freq.（%）	中标率 ASR China (1/10^5)	世标率 ASR World (1/10^5)	累积率 Cumulative rate(0~74, %)	顺位 Rank
全市 All areas	842	12.35	3.33	7.57	7.26	0.79	6
城区 Urban areas	544	12.86	3.22	7.85	7.49	0.83	8
郊区 Peri-urban areas	298	11.51	3.53	7.13	6.89	0.74	6

2017 年，北京市卵巢癌死亡病例数为 473 例，占女性全部恶性肿瘤死亡的 4.48%，位居女性恶性肿瘤死亡第 7 位；其中城区 318 例，郊区 155 例。卵巢癌死亡率为 6.94/10 万，中标死亡率为 3.44/10 万，世标死亡率为 3.38/10 万；城区世标死亡率为郊区的 1.14 倍。0~74 岁累积死亡率为 0.41%（表 5.15.2）。

A total of 473 cases died of ovarian cancer (318 in urban areas and 155 in peri-urban areas), accounting for 4.48% of all female cancer deaths in 2017. Ovarian cancer was the 7th leading cause of cancer deaths in all female cancers. The crude mortality rate was 6.94 per 100,000, with an ASR China and an ASR World of 3.44 and 3.38 per 100,000 respectively. The ASR World for mortality was 14% higher in urban areas than that in peri-urban areas. The cumulative mortality rate for subjects aged 0 to 74 years was 0.41% (Table 5.15.2).

表 5.15.2 2017 年北京市户籍居民卵巢癌死亡情况
Table 5.15.2 Mortality of ovarian cancer in Beijing, 2017

地区 Areas	例数 No. deaths	粗率 Crude rate (1/10^5)	构成比 Freq.（%）	中标率 ASR China (1/10^5)	世标率 ASR World (1/10^5)	累积率 Cumulative rate(0~74, %)	顺位 Rank
全市 All areas	473	6.94	4.48	3.44	3.38	0.41	7
城区 Urban areas	318	7.52	4.54	3.59	3.54	0.43	7
郊区 Peri-urban areas	155	5.99	4.37	3.16	3.11	0.37	8

北京市卵巢癌世标发病率由 2008 年的 6.23/10 万上升到 2017 年的 7.26/10 万，发病率年均变化百分比为 0.90%（P=0.162）。北京市卵巢癌世标死亡率由 2008 年的 3.11/10 万上升到 2017 年的 3.38/10 万，死亡率年均变化百分比为 1.10%（P=0.185）。

卵巢癌年龄别发病率在 35 岁以前处于较低水平，自 35~39 岁年龄组开始快速上升，至 70~74 岁年龄组达高峰（图 5.15.1）。卵巢癌年龄别死亡率在 30 岁之前处于较低水平，自 30~34 岁年龄组开始快速上升，至 75~79 岁年龄组达高峰（图 5.15.4）。城区和郊区年龄别发病率、死亡率变化有一定差别，但总体趋势相同，郊区波动较为明显（图 5.15.2 和图 5.15.3，图 5.15.5 和图 5.15.6）。

The ASR World for incidence of ovarian cancer increased from 6.23 per 100,000 in 2008 to 7.26 per 100,000 in 2017, the APC of ASR World for incidence was 0.90% (P=0.162). The ASR World for mortality of ovarian cancer increased from 3.11 per 100,000 in 2008 to 3.38 per 100,000 in 2017, the APC of ASR World for mortality was 1.10% (P=0.185).

The age-specific incidence rates of ovarian cancer were relatively low in people below 35 years old, and the rate increased sharply in people at the age group of 35-39 years, peaking at the age group of 70-74 years (Figure 5.15.1). The age-specific mortality rates of ovarian cancer were relatively low in people below 30 years old, and the rate increased sharply in people at the age group of 30-34 years, peaking at the age group of 75-79 years (Figure 5.15.4). There were some differences in age-specific incidence and mortality rates between urban and peri-urban areas, but the overall trends were same. The incidence and mortality rates in peri-urban areas showed huge fluctuations (Figure 5.15.2-5.15.3, Figure 5.15.5-5.15.6).

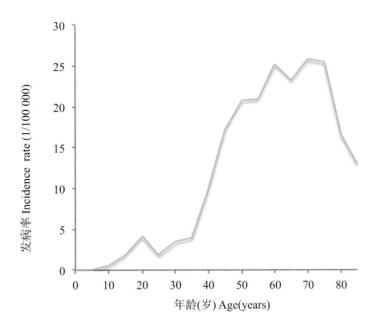

图 5.15.1 2017 年北京市户籍居民卵巢癌年龄别发病率
Figure 5.15.1 Age-specific incidence rate of ovarian cancer in Beijing, 2017

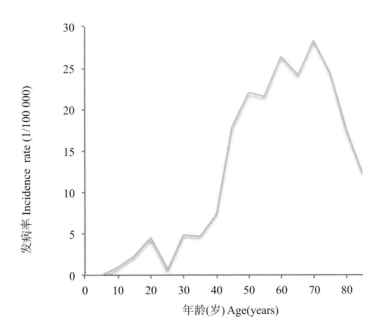

图 5.15.2 2017 年北京市城区户籍居民卵巢癌年龄别发病率
Figure 5.15.2 Age-specific incidence rate of ovarian cancer in urban areas of Beijing, 2017

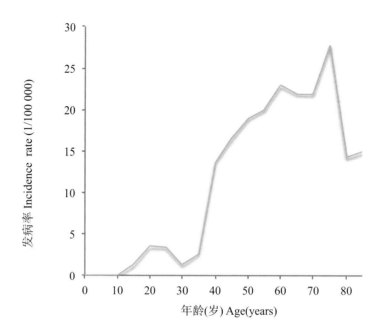

图 5.15.3 2017 年北京市郊区户籍居民卵巢癌年龄别发病率
Figure 5.15.3 Age-specific incidence rate of ovarian cancer in peri-urban areas of Beijing, 2017

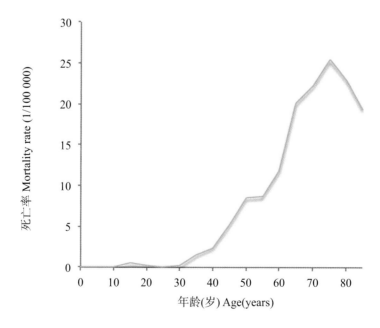

图 5.15.4 2017 年北京市户籍居民卵巢癌年龄别死亡率
Figure 5.15.4 Age-specific mortality rate of ovarian cancer in Beijing, 2017

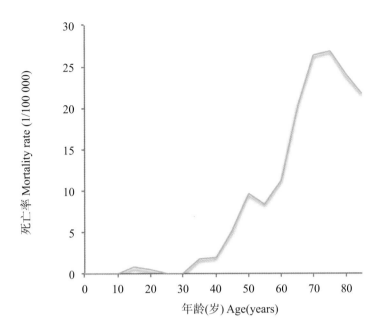

图 5.15.5 2017 年北京市城区户籍居民卵巢癌年龄别死亡率
Figure 5.15.5 Age-specific mortality rate of ovarian cancer in urban areas of Beijing, 2017

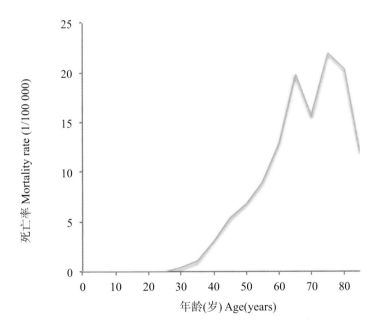

图 5.15.6 2017 年北京市郊区户籍居民卵巢癌年龄别死亡率
Figure 5.15.6 Age-specific mortality rate of ovarian cancer in peri-urban areas of Beijing, 2017

2017 年，北京市卵巢癌世标发病率和死亡率在 16 个辖区间有一定差异，城区发病率和死亡率均高于郊区（图 5.15.7 和图 5.15.8）。

In 2017, there were some differences between the 16 districts in ASR World for incidence and mortality of ovarian cancer in Beijing. The incidence and mortality rates of ovarian cancer were higher in urban areas than those in peri-urban areas (Figure 5.15.7-5.15.8).

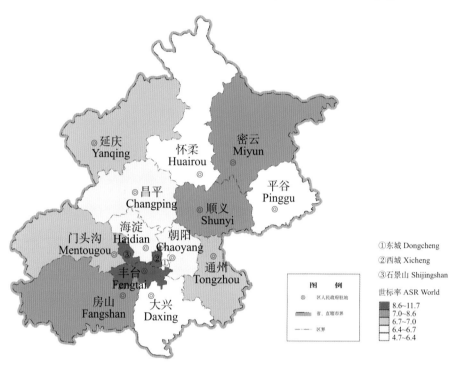

图 5.15.7 2017 年北京市户籍居民卵巢癌发病率（1/10^5）地区分布情况
Figure 5.15.7 Incidence rates of ovarian cancer by district in Beijing, 2017（1/10^5）

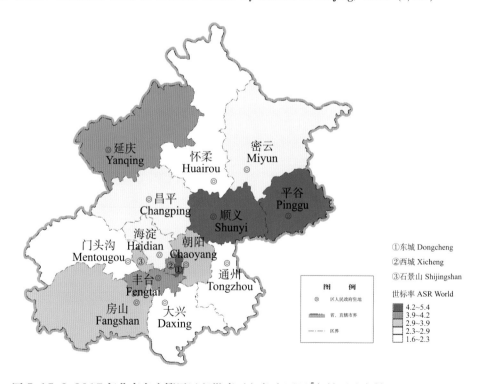

图 5.15.8 2017 年北京市户籍居民卵巢癌死亡率（1/10^5）地区分布情况
Figure 5.15.8 Mortality rates of ovarian cancer by district in Beijing, 2017（1/10^5）

（撰稿　张希，校稿　程杨杨）

5.16 前列腺 (C61)

2017 年，北京市前列腺癌新发病例数为 1 606 例，占男性全部恶性肿瘤发病的 6.49%，位居男性恶性肿瘤发病第 5 位；其中城区 1 187 例，郊区 419 例。前列腺癌发病率为 23.65/10 万，中标发病率为 10.50/10 万，世标发病率为 10.30/10 万；城区世标发病率为郊区的 1.47 倍。0~74 岁累积发病率为 1.31%（表 5.16.1）。

5.16 Prostate (C61)

There were 1,606 new cases diagnosed as prostate cancer (1,187 in urban areas and 419 in peri-urban areas), accounting for 6.49% of new cases of all male cancers in 2017. Prostate cancer was the 5th common male cancer in Beijing. The crude incidence rate was 23.65 per 100,000, with an ASR China and ASR World of 10.50 and 10.30 per 100,000, respectively. The ASR World for incidence was 47% higher in urban areas than in peri-urban areas. The cumulative incidence rate for subjects aged 0 to 74 years was 1.31% (Table 5.16.1).

表 5.16.1 2017 年北京市户籍居民前列腺癌发病情况
Table 5.16.1 Incidence of prostate cancer in Beijing, 2017

地区 Areas	例数 No. cases	粗率 Crude rate ($1/10^5$)	构成比 Freq.（%）	中标率 ASR China ($1/10^5$)	世标率 ASR World ($1/10^5$)	累积率 Cumulative rate(0~74, %)	顺位 Rank
全市 All areas	1 606	23.65	6.49	10.50	10.30	1.31	5
城区 Urban areas	1 187	28.20	7.37	11.94	11.72	1.55	3
郊区 Peri-urban areas	419	16.23	4.85	8.06	7.97	0.92	6

2017 年，北京市前列腺癌死亡病例数为 613 例，占男性全部恶性肿瘤死亡的 3.95%，位居男性恶性肿瘤死亡第 7 位；其中城区 455 例，郊区 158 例。前列腺癌死亡率为 9.03/10 万，中标死亡率为 3.06/10 万，世标死亡率为 3.03/10 万；城区世标死亡率为郊区的 1.14 倍。0~74 岁累积死亡率为 0.22%（表 5.16.2）。

A total of 613 cases died of prostate cancer (455 in urban areas and 158 in peri-urban areas), accounting for 3.95% of all male cancer deaths in 2017. Prostate cancer was the 7th leading cause of cancer deaths in all male cancers. The crude mortality rate was 9.03 per 100,000, with an ASR China and an ASR World of 3.06 and 3.03 per 100,000, respectively. The ASR World for mortality in urban areas was 14% higher than that in peri-urban areas. The cumulative mortality rate for subjects aged 0 to 74 years was 0.22% (Table 5.16.2).

表 5.16.2 2017 年北京市户籍居民前列腺癌死亡情况
Table 5.16.2 Mortality of prostate cancer in Beijing, 2017

地区 Areas	例数 No. deaths	粗率 Crude rate (1/10⁵)	构成比 Freq. (%)	中标率 ASR China (1/10⁵)	世标率 ASR World (1/10⁵)	累积率 Cumulative rate(0~74, %)	顺位 Rank
全市 All areas	613	9.03	3.95	3.06	3.03	0.22	7
城区 Urban areas	455	10.81	4.56	3.20	3.15	0.22	7
郊区 Peri-urban areas	158	6.12	2.86	2.77	2.76	0.21	11

北京市前列腺癌世标发病率由 2008 年的 7.05/10 万上升到 2017 年的 10.30/10 万，年均变化百分比为 3.94%（P=0.001）。前列腺癌世标死亡率由 2008 年的 2.51/10 万上升到 2017 年的 3.03/10 万，年均变化百分比为 1.23%（P=0.113）。

前列腺癌年龄别发病率和死亡率在 55 岁以前均较低，55 岁开始呈上升趋势，60 岁之后快速上升。城区和郊区发病率均在 75~79 岁组达到高峰，而死亡率均在 85 岁及以上年龄组达到高峰（图 5.16.1 至图 5.16.6）。

The ASR World for incidence of prostate cancer increased from 7.05 per 100,000 in 2008 to 10.30 per 100,000 in 2017; the APC of ASR World for incidence of prostate cancer was 3.94% (P=0.001). The ASR World for mortality increased from 2.51 per 100,000 in 2008 to 3.03 per 100,000 in 2017; the APC of ASR World for mortality was 1.23% (P =0.113).

The age-specific incidence and mortality rates of prostate cancer were low in men under 55 years old and increased constantly in older men. The age-specific incidence and mortality rates increased dramatically in men older than 60 years. The incidence and mortality rates in both urban and peri-urban areas peaked at the age groups of 75-79 years and 85 years and above, respectively (Figure 5.16.1-5.16.6).

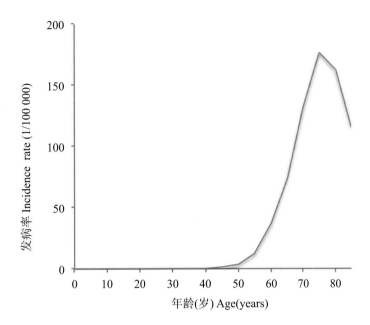

图 5.16.1 2017 年北京市户籍居民前列腺癌年龄别发病率
Figure 5.16.1 Age-specific incidence rate of prostate cancer in Beijing, 2017

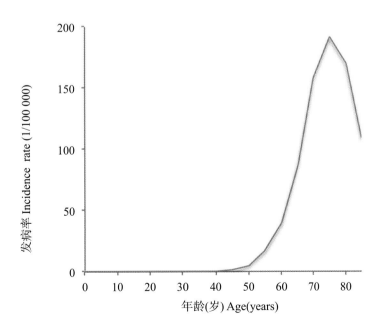

图 5.16.2 2017 年北京市城区户籍居民前列腺癌年龄别发病率
Figure 5.16.2 Age-specific incidence rate of prostate cancer in urban areas of Beijing, 2017

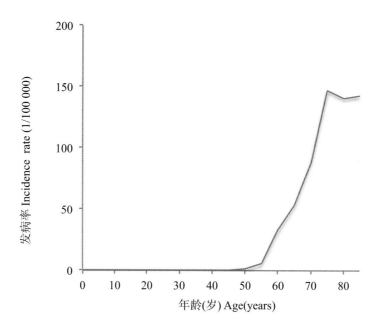

图 5.16.3 2017 年北京市郊区户籍居民前列腺癌年龄别发病率
Figure 5.16.3 Age-specific incidence rate of prostate cancer in peri-urban areas of Beijing, 2017

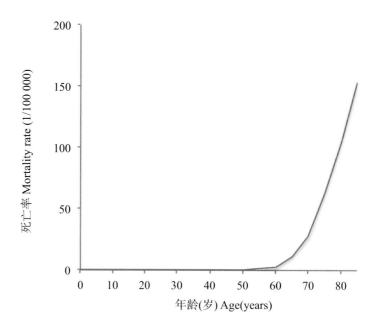

图 5.16.4 2017 年北京市户籍居民前列腺癌年龄别死亡率
Figure 5.16.4 Age-specific mortality rate of prostate cancer in Beijing, 2017

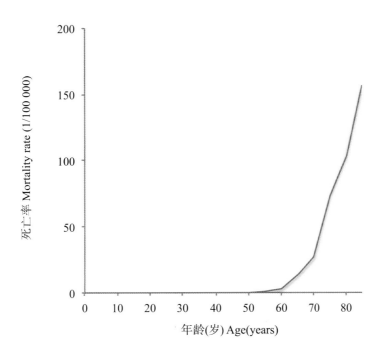

图 5.16.5 2017 年北京市城区户籍居民前列腺癌年龄别死亡率
Figure 5.16.5 Age-specific mortality rate of prostate cancer in urban areas of Beijing, 2017

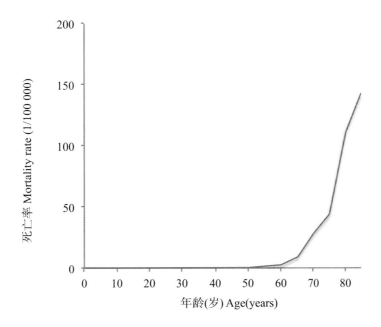

图 5.16.6 2017 年北京市郊区户籍居民前列腺癌年龄别死亡率
Figure 5.16.6 Age-specific mortality rate of prostate cancer in peri-urban areas of Beijing, 2017

2017 年，北京市前列腺癌世标发病率和死亡率在 16 个辖区间有一定差异，城区发病率和死亡率均高于郊区（图 5.16.7 和图 5.16.8）。

In 2017, There were some differences between the 16 districts in ASR World for incidence and mortality of prostate cancer in Beijing. The incidence and mortality rates were higher in urban areas than in peri-urban areas（Figure 5.16.7-5.16.8）.

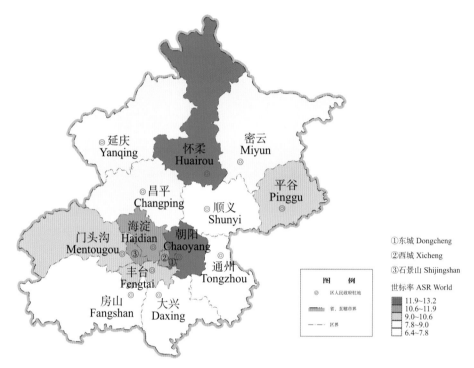

图 5.16.7 2017 年北京市户籍居民前列腺癌发病率（1/10⁵）地区分布情况
Figure 5.16.7 Incidence rates distribution of prostate cancer by district in Beijing, 2017(1/10⁵)

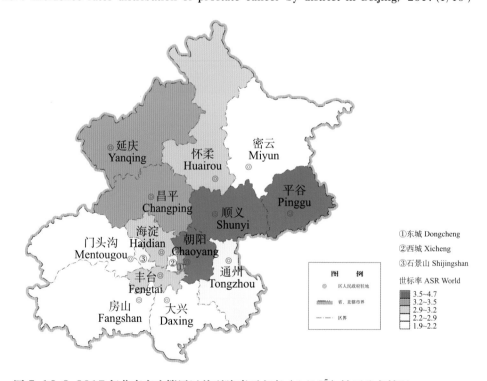

图 5.16.8 2017 年北京市户籍居民前列腺癌死亡率（1/10⁵）地区分布情况
Figure 5.16.8 Mortality rates of prostate cancer by district in Beijing, 2017(1/10⁵)

（撰稿 李慧超，校稿 刘硕）

5.17 肾及泌尿系统部位不明 (C64–66, C68)

2017 年，北京市肾及泌尿系统部位不明癌新发病例数为 2 092 例，占全部恶性肿瘤发病的 4.18%，位居恶性肿瘤发病第 9 位；其中男性 1 272 例，女性 820 例，城区 1 445 例，郊区 647 例。肾及泌尿系统部位不明癌发病率为 15.37/10 万，中标发病率为 8.03/10 万，世标发病率为 7.86/10 万；男性世标发病率为女性的 1.75 倍，城区世标发病率为郊区的 1.22 倍。0~74 岁累积发病率为 0.93%（表 5.17.1）。

5.17 Kidney & unspecified urinary organs (C64–66, C68)

There were 2,092 new cases diagnosed as cancer of kidney & unspecified urinary organs (1,272 males and 820 females, 1,445 in urban areas and 647 in peri-urban areas), accounting for 4.18% of new cases of all cancers in 2017. Cancer of kidney & unspecified urinary organs was the 9th common cancer in Beijing. The crude incidence rate was 15.37 per 100,000, with an ASR China and an ASR World of 8.03 and 7.86 per 100,000, respectively. The ASR World for incidence was 75% higher in males than in females and 22% higher in urban areas than in peri-urban areas, respectively. The cumulative incidence rate for subjects aged 0 to 74 years was 0.93% (Table 5.17.1).

表 5.17.1 2017 年北京市户籍居民肾及泌尿系统部位不明癌发病情况
Table 5.17.1 Incidence of Cancer of kidney & unspecified urinary organs in Beijing, 2017

地区 Areas	性别 Sex	例数 No. cases	粗率 Crude rate (1/10^5)	构成比 Freq.(%)	中标率 ASR China (1/10^5)	世标率 ASR World (1/10^5)	累积率 Cumulative rate(0~74, %)	顺位 Rank
全市 All areas	合计 Both	2 092	15.37	4.18	8.03	7.86	0.93	9
	男性 Male	1 272	18.73	5.14	10.32	10.03	1.20	6
	女性 Female	820	12.03	3.24	5.80	5.74	0.66	7
城区 Urban areas	合计 Both	1 445	17.12	4.38	8.63	8.42	0.99	9
	男性 Male	889	21.12	5.52	11.28	10.95	1.31	6
	女性 Female	556	13.14	3.29	6.03	5.94	0.68	7
郊区 Peri-urban areas	合计 Both	647	12.51	3.79	7.00	6.88	0.82	9
	男性 Male	383	14.83	4.43	8.70	8.46	1.02	9
	女性 Female	264	10.20	3.13	5.35	5.35	0.64	7

2017 年，北京市肾及泌尿系统部位不明癌死亡病例数为 751 例，占全部恶性肿瘤死亡的 2.88%，位居恶性肿瘤死亡第 13 位；其中男性 443 例，女性 308 例，城区 551 例，郊区 200 例。肾及泌尿系统部位不明癌死亡率为 5.52/10 万，中标死亡率为 2.13/10 万，世标死亡率为 2.15/10 万；男性世标死亡率为女性的 1.82 倍，城区世标死亡率为郊区的 1.25 倍。0~74 岁累积死亡率为 0.20%（表 5.17.2）。

A total of 751 cases died of cancer of kidney & unspecified urinary organs (443 males and 308 females, 551 in urban areas and 200 in peri-urban areas), accounting for 2.88% of all cancer deaths in 2017. Cancer of kidney & unspecified urinary organs was the 13th leading cause of cancer deaths in all kinds of cancer. The crude mortality rate was 5.52 per 100,000, with an ASR China and ASR World of 2.13 and 2.15 per 100,000, respectively. The ASR World for mortality was 82% higher in males than in females and 25% higher in urban areas than in peri-urban areas. The cumulative mortality rate for subjects aged 0 to 74 years was 0.20% (Table 5.17.2).

表 5.17.2 2017 年北京市户籍居民肾及泌尿系统部位不明癌死亡情况
Table 5.17.2 Mortality of Cancer of kidney & unspecified urinary organs in Beijing, 2017

地区 Areas	性别 Sex	例数 No. deaths	粗率 Crude rate （1/10^5）	构成比 Freq.（%）	中标率 ASR China （1/10^5）	世标率 ASR World （1/10^5）	累积率 Cumulative rate（0~74, %）	顺位 Rank
全市 All areas	合计 Both	751	5.52	2.88	2.13	2.15	0.20	13
	男性 Male	443	6.52	2.86	2.77	2.80	0.29	12
	女性 Female	308	4.52	2.92	1.52	1.54	0.12	11
城区 Urban areas	合计 Both	551	6.53	3.24	2.28	2.30	0.22	12
	男性 Male	321	7.63	3.22	3.01	3.04	0.34	11
	女性 Female	230	5.44	3.28	1.59	1.59	0.11	10
郊区 Peri-urban areas	合计 Both	200	3.87	2.21	1.82	1.85	0.18	15
	男性 Male	122	4.73	2.21	2.36	2.40	0.23	12
	女性 Female	78	3.01	2.20	1.32	1.34	0.13	13

按部位划分,肾癌(C64)发病率为11.11/10万,中标发病率为6.21/10万,世标发病率为6.07/10万;肾癌死亡率为3.28/10万,中标死亡率为1.35/10万,世标死亡率为1.39/10万。肾盂癌(C65)发病率为1.84/10万,中标发病率为0.79/10万,世标发病率为0.78/10万;肾盂癌死亡率为0.84/10万,中标死亡率为0.29/10万,世标死亡率为0.28/10万。输尿管癌(C66)发病率为1.96/10万,中标发病率为0.82/10万,世标发病率为0.81/10万;输尿管癌死亡率为1.14/10万,中标死亡率为0.40/10万,世标死亡率为0.39/10万(表5.17.3至表5.17.8)。

By subsite, the kidney cancer (C64) incidence rate was 11.11 per 100,000, with ASR China 6.21 per 100,000 and ASR World 6.07 per 100,000; and the mortality rate was 3.28 per 100,000, with ASR China 1.35 per 100,000 and ASR World 1.39 per 100,000. The incidence rate of renal pelvis cancer (C65) was 1.84 per 100,000, with ASR China 0.79 per 100,000 and ASR World 0.78 per 100,000; and the mortality rate was 0.84 per 100,000, with ASR China 0.29 per 100,000 and ASR World 0.28 per 100,000. The ureter cancer (C66) incidence rate was 1.96 per 100,000, with ASR China 0.82 per 100,000 and ASR World 0.81 per 100,000; and the mortality rate was 1.14 per 100,000, with ASR China 0.40 per 100,000 and ASR World 0.39 per 100,000 (Table 5.17.3-5.17.8).

表 5.17.3 2017 年北京市户籍居民肾癌(C64)发病情况
Table 5.17.3 Incidence of kidney cancer(C64) in Beijing, 2017

地区 Areas	性别 Sex	例数 No. cases	粗率 Crude rate (1/10⁵)	构成比 Freq.(%)	中标率 ASR China (1/10⁵)	世标率 ASR World (1/10⁵)	累积率 Cumulative rate(0~74,%)
全市 All areas	合计 Both	1 512	11.11	3.02	6.21	6.07	0.72
	男性 Male	1 002	14.75	4.05	8.50	8.22	0.98
	女性 Female	510	7.48	2.01	3.99	3.98	0.47
城区 Urban areas	合计 Both	1 048	12.42	3.18	6.77	6.61	0.78
	男性 Male	711	16.89	4.41	9.44	9.16	1.10
	女性 Female	337	7.97	2.00	4.14	4.11	0.48
郊区 Peri-urban areas	合计 Both	464	8.97	2.72	5.30	5.18	0.62
	男性 Male	291	11.27	3.37	6.92	6.64	0.79
	女性 Female	173	6.68	2.05	3.72	3.75	0.45

表 5.17.4　2017 年北京市户籍居民肾癌（C64）死亡情况
Table 5.17.4 Mortality of kidney cancer (C64) in Beijing, 2017

地区 Areas	性别 Sex	例数 No. deaths	粗率 Crude rate （1/10⁵）	构成比 Freq.（%）	中标率 ASR China （1/10⁵）	世标率 ASR World （1/10⁵）	累积率 Cumulative rate(0~74,%)
全市 All areas	合计 Both	446	3.28	1.71	1.35	1.39	0.14
	男性 Male	297	4.37	1.91	1.94	1.97	0.21
	女性 Female	149	2.19	1.41	0.79	0.85	0.08
城区 Urban areas	合计 Both	326	3.86	1.92	1.46	1.51	0.16
	男性 Male	219	5.20	2.19	2.15	2.19	0.24
	女性 Female	107	2.53	1.52	0.80	0.85	0.07
郊区 Peri-urban areas	合计 Both	120	2.32	1.32	1.13	1.17	0.12
	男性 Male	78	3.02	1.41	1.57	1.56	0.15
	女性 Female	42	1.62	1.18	0.72	0.80	0.08

表 5.17.5　2017 年北京市户籍居民肾盂癌（C65）发病情况
Table 5.17.5 Incidence of renal pelvis cancer (C65) in Beijing, 2017

地区 Areas	性别 Sex	例数 No. cases	粗率 Crude rate （1/10⁵）	构成比 Freq.（%）	中标率 ASR China （1/10⁵）	世标率 ASR World （1/10⁵）	累积率 Cumulative rate(0~74,%)
全市 All areas	合计 Both	251	1.84	0.50	0.79	0.78	0.09
	男性 Male	113	1.66	0.46	0.76	0.76	0.09
	女性 Female	138	2.02	0.55	0.81	0.79	0.09
城区 Urban areas	合计 Both	179	2.12	0.54	0.85	0.84	0.10
	男性 Male	78	1.85	0.48	0.80	0.80	0.10
	女性 Female	101	2.39	0.60	0.89	0.87	0.11
郊区 Peri-urban areas	合计 Both	72	1.39	0.42	0.67	0.66	0.08
	男性 Male	35	1.36	0.41	0.68	0.68	0.08
	女性 Female	37	1.43	0.44	0.66	0.64	0.07

表 5.17.6 2017 年北京市户籍居民肾盂癌（C65）死亡情况
Table 5.17.6 Mortality of renal pelvis cancer(C65) in Beijing, 2017

地区 Areas	性别 Sex	例数 No. deaths	粗率 Crude rate （1/10⁵）	构成比 Freq.（%）	中标率 ASR China （1/10⁵）	世标率 ASR World （1/10⁵）	累积率 Cumulative rate(0~74, %)
全市 All areas	合计 Both	115	0.84	0.44	0.29	0.28	0.02
	男性 Male	54	0.80	0.35	0.30	0.30	0.03
	女性 Female	61	0.89	0.58	0.27	0.25	0.01
城区 Urban areas	合计 Both	82	0.97	0.48	0.28	0.28	0.02
	男性 Male	37	0.88	0.37	0.28	0.29	0.03
	女性 Female	45	1.06	0.64	0.28	0.26	0.01
郊区 Peri-urban areas	合计 Both	33	0.64	0.36	0.29	0.27	0.02
	男性 Male	17	0.66	0.31	0.33	0.32	0.03
	女性 Female	16	0.62	0.45	0.26	0.22	0.01

表 5.17.7 2017 年北京市户籍居民输尿管癌（C66）发病情况
Table 5.17.7 Incidence of ureter cancer(C66) in Beijing, 2017

地区 Areas	性别 Sex	例数 No. cases	粗率 Crude rate （1/10⁵）	构成比 Freq.（%）	中标率 ASR China （1/10⁵）	世标率 ASR World （1/10⁵）	累积率 Cumulative rate(0~74, %)
全市 All areas	合计 Both	267	1.96	0.53	0.82	0.81	0.09
	男性 Male	120	1.77	0.48	0.81	0.80	0.10
	女性 Female	147	2.16	0.58	0.84	0.81	0.08
城区 Urban areas	合计 Both	174	2.06	0.53	0.80	0.77	0.08
	男性 Male	71	1.69	0.44	0.74	0.72	0.09
	女性 Female	103	2.43	0.61	0.85	0.81	0.08
郊区 Peri-urban areas	合计 Both	93	1.80	0.54	0.86	0.86	0.10
	男性 Male	49	1.90	0.57	0.93	0.97	0.11
	女性 Female	44	1.70	0.52	0.79	0.77	0.09

表 5.17.8 2017 年北京市户籍居民输尿管癌（C66）死亡情况
Table 5.17.8 Mortality of ureter cancer (C66) in Beijing, 2017

地区 Areas	性别 Sex	例数 No. deaths	粗率 Crude rate (1/10⁵)	构成比 Freq.（%）	中标率 ASR China (1/10⁵)	世标率 ASR World (1/10⁵)	累积率 Cumulative rate(0~74, %)
全市 All areas	合计 Both	155	1.14	0.60	0.40	0.39	0.03
	男性 Male	70	1.03	0.45	0.41	0.41	0.04
	女性 Female	85	1.25	0.81	0.40	0.38	0.03
城区 Urban areas	合计 Both	115	1.36	0.68	0.43	0.41	0.03
	男性 Male	49	1.16	0.49	0.44	0.42	0.05
	女性 Female	66	1.56	0.94	0.42	0.39	0.02
郊区 Peri-urban areas	合计 Both	40	0.77	0.44	0.34	0.36	0.04
	男性 Male	21	0.81	0.38	0.37	0.41	0.04
	女性 Female	19	0.73	0.54	0.32	0.32	0.03

北京市肾及泌尿系统部位不明癌世标发病率由 2008 年的 6.53/10 万上升到 2017 年的 7.86/10 万，年均变化百分比为 2.31%（P<0.001）；男性和女性发病 10 年间年均变化百分比分别为 2.68%（P<0.001）和 1.68%（P=0.029）。北京市肾及泌尿系统部位不明癌世标死亡率由 2008 年的 1.75/10 万上升到 2017 年的 2.15/10 万，年均变化百分比为 0.67%（P=0.482）；男性和女性死亡 10 年间年均变化百分比分别为 0.32%（P=0.800）和 1.11%（P=0.229）。

肾及泌尿系统部位不明癌年龄别发病率在 30 岁之前均处于较低水平，自 30~34 岁组开始快速上升，至 75~79 岁组达到高峰，80~84 岁组以后降低；年龄别死亡率自 55~59 岁组开始快速上升。

The ASR World for incidence rate of cancer of kidney & unspecified urinary organs increased from 6.53 per 100,000 in 2008 to 7.86 per 100,000 in 2017; the APC of ASR World for incidence was 2.31% (P<0.001). The APCs of ASR World for incidence of cancer of kidney & unspecified urinary organs in males and females were 2.68% (P<0.001) and 1.68% (P=0.029), respectively. The ASR World for mortality of cancer of kidney & unspecified urinary organs increased from 1.75 per 100,000 in 2008 to 2.15 per 100,000 in 2017; the APC of ASR World for mortality was 0.67% (P=0.482). The APCs of ASR World for mortality of cancer of kidney & unspecified urinary organs in males and females were 0.32% (P=0.800) and 1.11% (P=0.229), respectively.

The age-specific incidence of cancer of kidney & unspecified urinary organs was at low levels in age below 30 years, and thereafter increased rapidly, peaking at the age group of 75-79 years, and declining at the age group of 80-84 years. Age-specific mortality rate increased rapidly in the age group older than 55 years. Age-specific incidence rates at the age groups

20~84 岁组各年龄别发病率和 20~74 岁组各年龄别死亡率均为男性明显高于女性（图 5.17.1 至图 5.17.6）

of 20-84 years and mortality rates at the age groups of 20-74 years in males were generally higher than those in females (Figure 5.17.1-5.17.6).

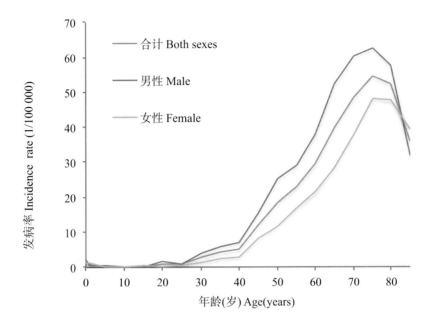

图 5.17.1 2017 年北京市户籍居民肾及泌尿系统部位不明癌年龄别发病率
Figure 5.17.1 Age-specific incidence rates of cancer of kidney & unspecified urinary organs in Beijing, 2017

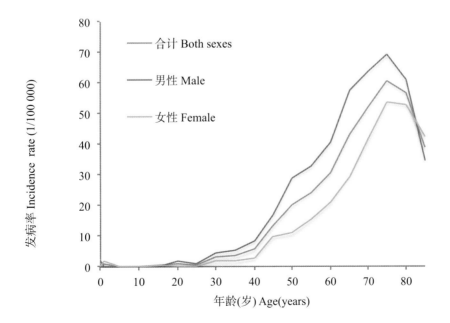

图 5.17.2 2017 年北京市城区户籍居民肾及泌尿系统部位不明癌年龄别发病率
Figure 5.17.2 Age-specific incidence rates of cancer of kidney & unspecified urinary organs in urban areas of Beijing, 2017

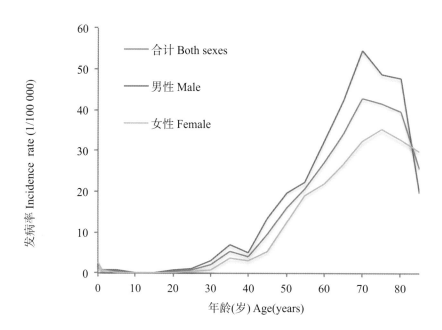

图 5.17.3 2017 年北京市郊区户籍居民肾及泌尿系统部位不明癌年龄别发病率
Figure 5.17.3 Age-specific incidence rates of cancer of kidney & unspecified urinary organs in peri-urban areas of Beijing, 2017

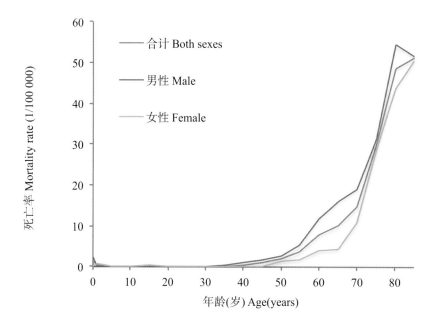

图 5.17.4 2017 年北京市户籍居民肾及泌尿系统部位不明癌年龄别死亡率
Figure 5.17.4 Age-specific mortality rates of cancer of kidney & unspecified urinary organs in Beijing, 2017

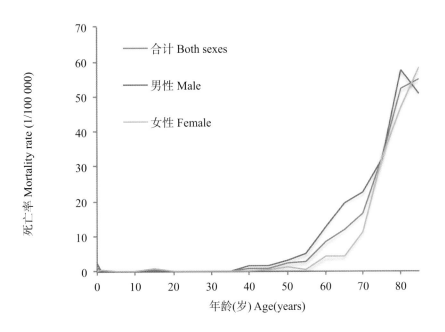

图 5.17.5 2017 年北京市城区户籍居民肾及泌尿系统部位不明癌年龄别死亡率
Figure 5.17.5 Age-specific mortality rates of cancer of kidney & unspecified urinary organs in urban areas of Beijing, 2017

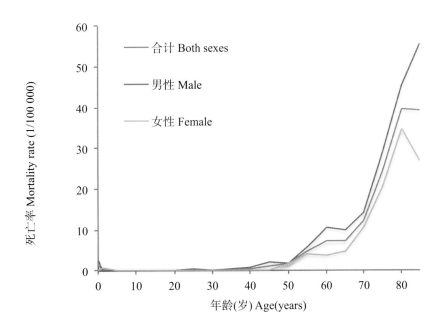

图 5.17.6 2017 年北京市郊区户籍居民肾及泌尿系统部位不明癌年龄别死亡率
Figure 5.17.6 Age-specific mortality rates of cancer of kidney & unspecified urinary organs in peri-urban areas of Beijing, 2017

2017 年，北京市肾及泌尿系统部位不明癌世标发病率和死亡率在 16 个辖区间有一定差异，城区发病率和死亡率均高于郊区（图 5.17.7 和图 5.17.8）。

In 2017, there were some differences between the 16 districts in ASR World for incidence and mortality in cancer of kidney & unspecified urinary organs in Beijing. The incidence and mortality rates were higher in urban areas than in peri-urban areas (Figure 5.17.7-5.17.8).

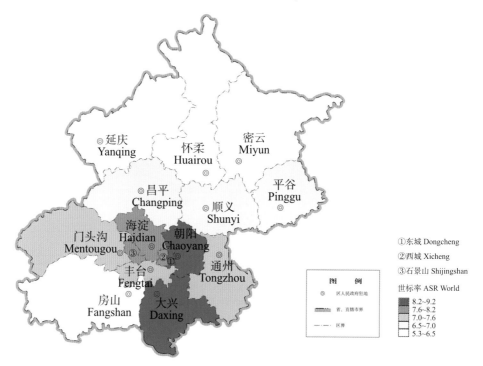

图 5.17.7 2017 年北京市户籍居民肾及泌尿系统部位不明癌发病率（1/10⁵）地区分布情况
Figure 5.17.7 Incidence rates of cancer of kidney & unspecified urinary organs by district of Beijing, 2017 (1/10⁵)

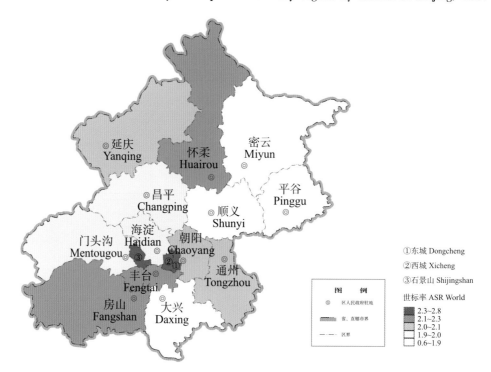

图 5.17.8 2017 年北京市户籍居民肾及泌尿系统部位不明癌死亡率（1/10⁵）地区分布情况
Figure 5.17.8 Mortality rates of cancer of kidney & unspecified urinary organs by district in Beijing, 2017 (1/10⁵)

肾（除外肾盂）是肾及泌尿系统部位不明癌发生的最主要亚部位，占全部病例的 72.28%，其次为输尿管，占 12.76%；肾盂占 12.00%；其他泌尿器官占 2.96%（图 5.17.9）

Kidney(except renal pelvis) was the most common subsite of cancer of kidney & unspecified urinary organs, accounting for 72.28% of all cases, followed by ureter (12.76%), renal pelvis (12.00%), and the other urinary organs (2.96%) (Figure 5.17.9).

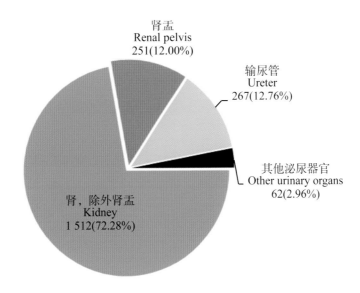

图 5.17.9 2017 年北京市户籍居民肾及泌尿系统部位不明癌亚部位分布情况

Figure 5.17.9 Subsite distribution of cancer of kidney & unspecified urinary organs in Beijing, 2017

（撰稿 李慧超，校稿 刘硕）

5.18 膀胱 (C67)

2017 年，北京市膀胱癌新发病例数为 1 727 例，占全部恶性肿瘤发病的 3.45%，位居恶性肿瘤发病第 10 位；其中男性 1 257 例，女性 470 例，城区 1 196 例，郊区 531 例。膀胱癌发病率为 12.69/10 万，中标发病率为 5.63/10 万，世标发病率为 5.58/10 万；男性世标发病率为女性的 2.89 倍，城区世标发病率为郊区的 1.13 倍。0~74 岁累积发病率为 0.66%（表 5.18.1）。

5.18 Bladder (C67)

There were 1,727 new cases diagnosed as bladder cancer (1,257 males and 470 females, 1,196 in urban areas and 531 in peri-urban areas), accounting for 3.45% of new cases of all cancers in 2017. Bladder cancer was the 10th common cancer in Beijing. The crude incidence rate was 12.69 per 100,000, with an ASR China and an ASR World of 5.63 and 5.58 per 100,000, respectively. The ASR World for incidence was 189% higher in males than in females and 13% higher in urban areas than in peri-urban areas. The cumulative incidence rate for subjects aged 0 to 74 years was 0.66% (Table 5.18.1).

表 5.18.1 2017 年北京市户籍居民膀胱癌发病情况
Table 5.18.1 Incidence of bladder cancer in Beijing, 2017

地区 Areas	性别 Sex	例数 No. cases	粗率 Crude rate (1/10⁵)	构成比 Freq.（%）	中标率 ASR China (1/10⁵)	世标率 ASR World (1/10⁵)	累积率 Cumulative rate(0~74, %)	顺位 Rank
全市 All areas	合计 Both	1 727	12.69	3.45	5.63	5.58	0.66	10
	男性 Male	1 257	18.51	5.08	8.51	8.44	0.99	7
	女性 Female	470	6.89	1.86	2.96	2.92	0.35	15
城区 Urban areas	合计 Both	1 196	14.17	3.62	5.86	5.80	0.69	10
	男性 Male	865	20.55	5.37	8.85	8.75	1.03	7
	女性 Female	331	7.82	1.96	3.07	3.03	0.36	13
郊区 Peri-urban areas	合计 Both	531	10.27	3.11	5.19	5.15	0.62	11
	男性 Male	392	15.18	4.54	7.92	7.89	0.93	7
	女性 Female	139	5.37	1.65	2.68	2.64	0.34	15

2017 年，北京市膀胱癌死亡病例数为 715 例，占全部恶性肿瘤死亡的 2.75%，位居恶性肿瘤死亡第 14 位；其中男性 524 例，女性 191 例，城区 494 例，郊区 221 例。膀胱癌死亡率为 5.25/10 万，

A total of 715 cases died of bladder cancer (524 males and 191 females, 494 in urban areas and 221 in peri-urban areas), accounting for 2.75% of all cancer deaths in 2017. Bladder cancer was the 14th leading cause of cancer deaths in all cancers. The crude mortality rate was 5.25 per 100,000, with an

中标死亡率为 1.69/10 万，世标死亡率为 1.72/10 万；男性世标死亡率为女性的 3.17 倍，郊区世标死亡率为城区的 1.14 倍。0~74 岁累积死亡率为 0.13%（表 5.18.2）。

ASR China and an ASR World of 1.69 and 1.72 per 100,000, respectively. The ASR World for mortality was 217% higher in males than in females and 14% higher in peri-urban areas than in urban areas. The cumulative mortality rate for subjects aged 0 to 74 years was 0.13% (Table 5.18.2).

表 5.18.2 2017 年北京市户籍居民膀胱癌死亡情况
Table 5.18.2 Mortality of bladder cancer in Beijing, 2017

地区 Areas	性别 Sex	例数 No. deaths	粗率 Crude rate （1/10⁵）	构成比 Freq.（%）	中标率 ASR China （1/10⁵）	世标率 ASR World （1/10⁵）	累积率 Cumulative rate(0~74, %)	顺位 Rank
全市 All areas	合计 Both	715	5.25	2.75	1.69	1.72	0.13	14
	男性 Male	524	7.72	3.38	2.64	2.69	0.21	9
	女性 Female	191	2.80	1.81	0.85	0.85	0.06	16
城区 Urban areas	合计 Both	494	5.85	2.91	1.58	1.63	0.12	13
	男性 Male	356	8.46	3.57	2.42	2.51	0.19	8
	女性 Female	138	3.26	1.97	0.83	0.82	0.06	15
郊区 Peri-urban areas	合计 Both	221	4.27	2.44	1.88	1.86	0.15	13
	男性 Male	168	6.51	3.04	3.04	3.03	0.24	10
	女性 Female	53	2.05	1.50	0.85	0.85	0.07	16

北京市膀胱癌世标发病率由 2008 年的 5.40/10 万上升到 2017 年的 5.58/10 万，年均变化百分比为 0.68%（P=0.126）；男性和女性发病 10 年间年均变化百分比分别为 0.78%（P=0.097）和 0.27%（P=0.730）。北京市膀胱癌世标死亡率由 2008 年的 1.65/10 万上升到 2017 年的 1.72/10 万，年均变化百分比为 -0.31%

The ASR World for incidence of bladder cancer increased from 5.40 per 100,000 in 2008 to 5.58 per 100,000 in 2017; the APC of ASR World for incidence was 0.68% (P=0.126).The APCs of ASR World for incidence of bladder cancer in males and females were 0.78% (P=0.097) and 0.27% (P=0.730), respectively. The ASR World for mortality of bladder cancer increased from 1.65 per 100,000 in 2008 to 1.72 per 100,000 in 2017; the APC of ASR World for mortality was -0.31% (P=0.599). The APCs of ASR World for

（P=0.599）；男性和女性死亡 10 年间年均变化百分比分别为 0.00%（P=0.999）和 −1.32%（P=0.179）。

膀胱癌年龄别发病率和死亡率呈现明显的性别差异。男性发病率自 50~54 岁组开始快速上升，至 80~84 岁组达到高峰（113.18/10 万）；女性发病率自 55~59 岁组开始上升，至 80~84 岁组达到高峰（41.13/10 万）。男性死亡率自 65~69 岁组开始快速上升，至 85 岁及以上组达到高峰（142.46/10 万）；女性死亡率自 70~74 岁组开始快速上升，至 85 岁及以上组达到高峰（40.80/10 万）。除 45 岁以下年龄组略有波动外，男性发病率和死亡率均高于女性（图 5.18.1 至图 5.18.6）。

mortality of bladder cancer in males and females were 0.00% (P=0.999) and −1.32% (P=0.179), respectively.

The trends of age-specific incidence and mortality rates showed differences between males and females in Beijing. The incidence rate in males increased rapidly from the age group of 50-54 years and peaked at the age group of 80-84 years (113.18 per 100,000). The incidence rate in females increased from the age group of 55-59 years and peaked at the age group of 80-84 years (41.13 per 100,000). The mortality rates in males and in females increased rapidly from the age group of 65-69 years and 70-74 years, respectively. Both sexes peaked at the age group of 85 years and above (males 142.46 per 100,000, females 40.80 per 100,000). Except for some fluctuation before 45 years old, the age-specific incidence and mortality rates for males were consistently higher than those for females (Figure 5.18.1-5.18.6).

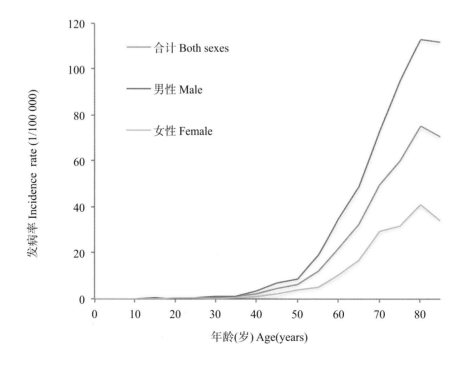

图 5.18.1 2017 年北京市户籍居民膀胱癌年龄别发病率
Figure 5.18.1 Age-specific incidence rates of bladder cancer in Beijing, 2017

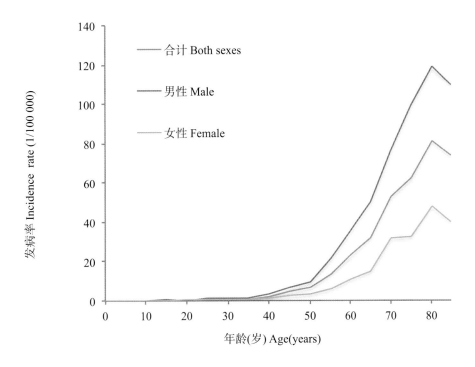

图 5.18.2 2017 年北京市城区户籍居民膀胱癌年龄别发病率
Figure 5.18.2 Age-specific incidence rates of bladder cancer in urban areas of Beijing, 2017

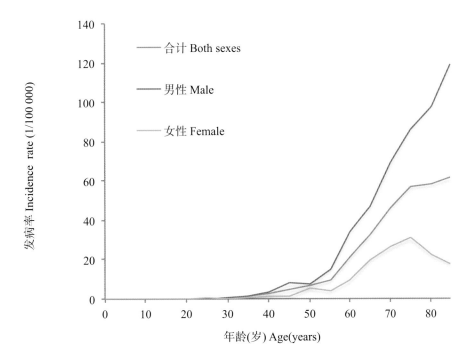

图 5.18.3 2017 年北京市郊区户籍居民膀胱癌年龄别发病率
Figure 5.18.3 Age-specific incidence rates of bladder cancer in peri-urban areas of Beijing, 2017

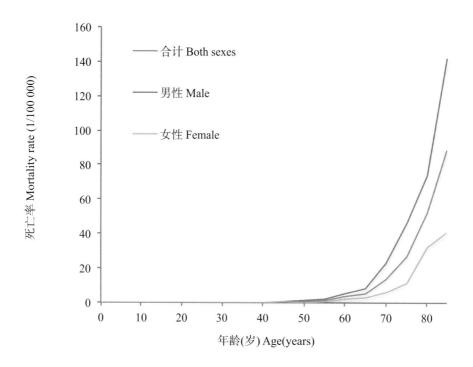

图 5.18.4 2017 年北京市户籍居民膀胱癌年龄别死亡率
Figure 5.18.4 Age-specific mortality rates of bladder cancer in Beijing, 2017

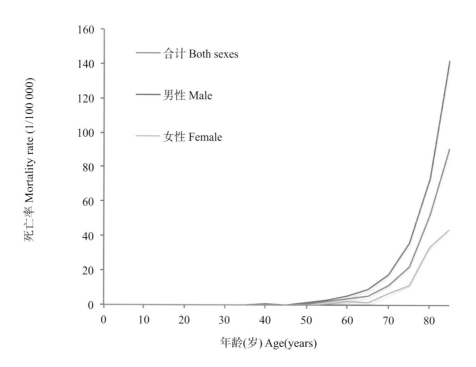

图 5.18.5 2017 年北京市城区户籍居民膀胱癌年龄别死亡率
Figure 5.18.5 Age-specific mortality rates of bladder cancer in urban areas of Beijing, 2017

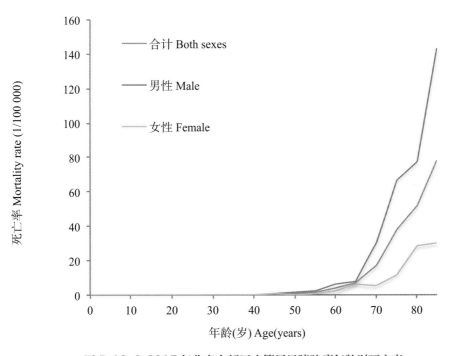

图 5.18.6　2017 年北京市郊区户籍居民膀胱癌年龄别死亡率

Figure 5.18.6　Age-specific mortality rates of bladder cancer in peri-urban areas of Beijing, 2017

2017 年，北京市膀胱癌世标发病率和死亡率在 16 个辖区间有一定差异，城区发病率高于郊区，郊区死亡率高于城区（图 5.18.7 和图 5.18.8 ）。

In 2017, There were some differences between the 16 districts in ASR World for incidence and mortality of bladder cancer in Beijing. The incidence rate was higher in urban areas than in peri-urban areas, while the mortality rate was higher in peri-urban areas than in urban areas（Figure 5.18.7-5.18.8 ）.

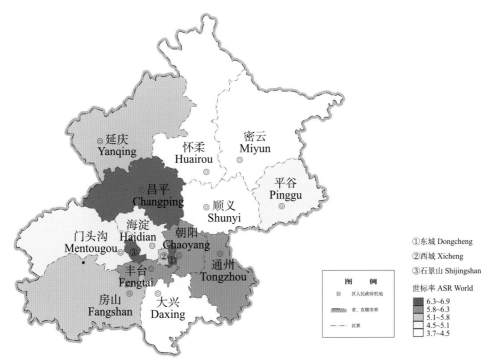

图 5.18.7　2017 年北京市户籍居民膀胱癌发病率（1/10^5）地区分布情况

Figure 5.18.7 Incidence rates of bladder cancer by district in Beijing, 2017(1/10^5)

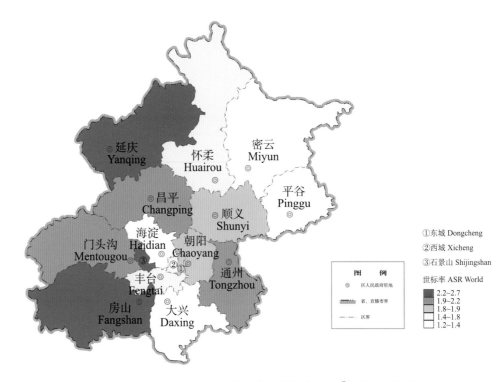

图 5.18.8 2017 年北京市户籍居民膀胱癌死亡率（1/10⁵）地区分布情况

Figure 5.18.8 Mortality rates of bladder cancer by district in Beijing, 2017(1/10⁵)

全部膀胱癌新发病例中，有明确亚部位的病例数占 31.67%，其中膀胱侧壁占 40.04%，膀胱后壁占 20.11%，输尿管口占 11.88%，膀胱三角区占 8.96%，膀胱前壁占 8.59%，膀胱顶占 4.75%，膀胱颈占 4.39%，脐尿管占 1.10%（图 5.18.9）。

About 31.67% cases were assigned to specified categories of bladder cancer sites. Among those, 40.04% of cases occurred in the lateral wall of bladder, followed by the posterior wall of bladder (20.11%), ureteric orifice (11.88%), the trigone (8.96%), the anterior wall of bladder (8.59%), the dome (4.75%), bladder neck (4.39%) and urachus (1.10%) (Figure 5.18.9).

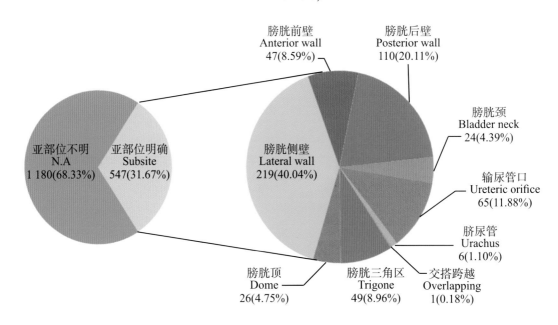

图 5.18.9 2017 年北京市户籍居民膀胱癌亚部位分布情况

Figure 5.18.9 Subsite distribution of bladder cancer in Beijing, 2017

（撰稿 李慧超，校稿 刘硕）

5.19 脑 (C70-72)

2017 年，北京市脑癌新发病例数为 666 例，占全部恶性肿瘤发病的 1.33%，位居恶性肿瘤发病第 18 位；其中男性 346 例，女性 320 例，城区 400 例，郊区 266 例。脑癌发病率为 4.89/10 万，中标发病率为 3.42/10 万，世标发病率为 3.34/10 万；男性世标发病率为女性的 1.19 倍，郊区世标发病率为城区的 1.11 倍。0~74 岁累积发病率为 0.30%（表 5.19.1）。

5.19 Brain (C70-72)

There were 666 new cases diagnosed as brain cancer (346 males and 320 females, 400 in urban areas and 266 in peri-urban areas), accounting for 1.33% of new cases of all cancers in 2017. Brain cancer was the 18th common cancer in Beijing. The crude incidence rate was 4.89 per 100,000, with an ASR China and an ASR World of 3.42 and 3.34 per 100,000, respectively. The ASR World for incidence was 19% higher in males than in females and 11% higher in peri-urban areas than in urban areas. The cumulative incidence rate for subjects aged 0 to 74 years was 0.30% (Table 5.19.1).

表 5.19.1 2017 年北京市户籍居民脑癌发病情况
Table 5.19.1 Incidence of brain cancer in Beijing, 2017

地区 Areas	性别 Sex	例数 No. cases	粗率 Crude rate (1/10⁵)	构成比 Freq.（%）	中标率 ASR China (1/10⁵)	世标率 ASR World (1/10⁵)	累积率 Cumulative rate(0~74, %)	顺位 Rank
全市 All areas	合计 Both	666	4.89	1.33	3.42	3.34	0.30	18
	男性 Male	346	5.09	1.40	3.76	3.63	0.34	15
	女性 Female	320	4.69	1.26	3.07	3.06	0.27	16
城区 Urban areas	合计 Both	400	4.74	1.21	3.27	3.24	0.30	19
	男性 Male	199	4.73	1.24	3.40	3.34	0.31	15
	女性 Female	201	4.75	1.19	3.12	3.13	0.28	16
郊区 Peri-urban areas	合计 Both	266	5.15	1.56	3.73	3.58	0.32	18
	男性 Male	147	5.69	1.70	4.39	4.15	0.39	14
	女性 Female	119	4.60	1.41	3.08	3.01	0.26	16

2017 年，北京市脑癌死亡病例数为 497 例，占全部恶性肿瘤死亡的 1.91%，位居恶性肿瘤死亡第 15 位；其中男性 243 例，女性 254 例，城区 296 例，郊区 201 例。脑癌死亡率为 3.65/10 万，

A total of 497 cases died of brain cancer (243 males and 254 females, 296 in urban areas and 201 in peri-urban areas), accounting for 1.91% of all cancer deaths in 2017. Brain cancer was the 15th leading cause of cancer deaths in all cancers. The crude mortality rate was 3.65 per 100,000, with an ASR China and an ASR

中标死亡率为 2.09/10 万，世标死亡率为 2.02/10 万；男性世标死亡率为女性的 1.04 倍，郊区世标死亡率为城区的 1.19 倍。0~74 岁累积死亡率为 0.21%（表 5.19.2）。

World of 2.09 and 2.02 per 100,000, respectively. The ASR World for mortality was 4% higher in males than in females and 19% higher in peri-urban areas than in urban areas. The cumulative mortality rate for subjects aged 0 to 74 years was 0.21% (Table 5.19.2).

表 5.19.2　2017 年北京市户籍居民脑癌死亡情况
Table 5.19.2 Mortality of brain cancer in Beijing, 2017

地区 Areas	性别 Sex	例数 No. deaths	粗率 Crude rate (1/10⁵)	构成比 Freq.（%）	中标率 ASR China (1/10⁵)	世标率 ASR World (1/10⁵)	累积率 Cumulative rate(0~74, %)	顺位 Rank
全市 All areas	合计 Both	497	3.65	1.91	2.09	2.02	0.21	15
	男性 Male	243	3.58	1.57	2.13	2.06	0.21	13
	女性 Female	254	3.73	2.41	2.04	1.98	0.20	12
城区 Urban areas	合计 Both	296	3.51	1.74	1.93	1.89	0.19	16
	男性 Male	138	3.28	1.38	1.81	1.78	0.18	14
	女性 Female	158	3.73	2.26	2.05	2.00	0.21	13
郊区 Peri-urban areas	合计 Both	201	3.89	2.22	2.36	2.25	0.23	14
	男性 Male	105	4.07	1.90	2.65	2.55	0.27	13
	女性 Female	96	3.71	2.71	2.06	1.95	0.20	12

北京市脑癌世标发病率由 2008 年的 3.68/10 万下降到 2017 年的 3.34/10 万，年均变化百分比为 -0.93%（P=0.068）；男性和女性发病 10 年间年均变化百分比分别为 -0.78%（P=0.190）和 -1.13%（P=0.218）。北京市脑癌世标死亡率由 2008 年的 2.48/10 万下降到 2017 年的 2.02/10 万，

The incidence of ASR World of brain cancer decreased from 3.68 per 100,000 in 2008 to 3.34 per 100,000 in 2017; the APC of ASR World for incidence was -0.93% (P=0.068). The APCs of ASR World for incidence of brain cancer in males and females were -0.78% (P=0.190) and -1.13% (P=0.218), respectively. The mortality of ASR World of brain cancer decreased from 2.48 per 100,000 in 2008 to 2.02 per 100,000 in 2017; the APC of ASR World for mortality was -0.99%

年均变化百分比为 -0.99%（*P*=0.299）；男性和女性死亡 10 年间年均变化百分比分别为 -0.65%（*P*=0.573）和 -1.45%（*P*=0.271）。

　　脑癌年龄别发病率和死亡率在 40 岁以前均较低，40 岁以后快速上升（图 5.19.1 至图 5.19.6）。不同性别发病率和死亡率变化无明显差异，男性的发病率和死亡率均在 80~84 岁组达到高峰，女性均在 75~79 岁组达到高峰（图 5.19.1 和图 5.19.4）。城区和郊区年龄别发病率、死亡率变化有一定差别，但总体趋势相同，郊区波动较为明显（图 5.19.2 和图 5.19.3，图 5.19.5 和图 5.19.6）。

(*P*=0.299). The APCs of ASR World for mortality of brain cancer in males and females were -0.65% (*P*=0.573) and -1.45% (*P*=0.271), respectively.

　　The age-specific incidence and mortality rates of brain cancer were relatively low in people below 40 years old, and the rates increased sharply in people older than that (Figure 5.19.1-5.19.6). There was no significant difference in incidence and mortality rates between males and females. The age-specific incidence and mortality rates for males peaked at the age group of 80-84 years, but at the age group of 75-79 years for females (Figure 5.19.1, Figure 5.19.4). There were some differences in age-specific incidence and mortality rates between urban and peri-urban areas, but the overall trends were same. The age-specific incidence and mortality rates in peri-urban areas showed huge fluctuations (Figure 5.19.2-5.19.3, Figure 5.19.5-5.19.6).

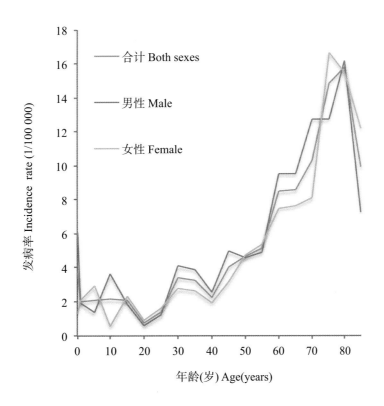

图 5.19.1 2017 年北京市户籍居民脑癌年龄别发病率
Figure 5.19.1 Age-specific incidence rates of brain cancer in Beijing, 2017

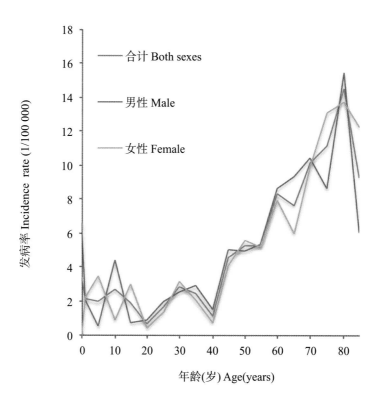

图 5.19.2 2017 年北京市城区户籍居民脑癌年龄别发病率
Figure 5.19.2 Age-specific incidence rates of brain cancer in urban areas of Beijing, 2017

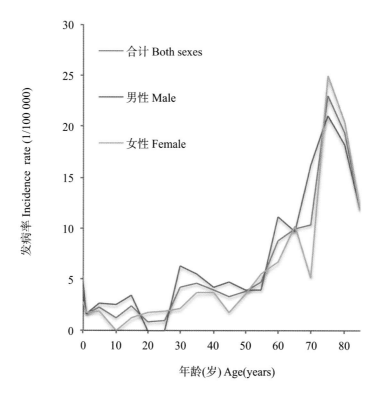

图 5.19.3 2017 年北京市郊区户籍居民脑癌年龄别发病率
Figure 5.19.3 Age-specific incidence rates of brain cancer in peri-urban areas of Beijing, 2017

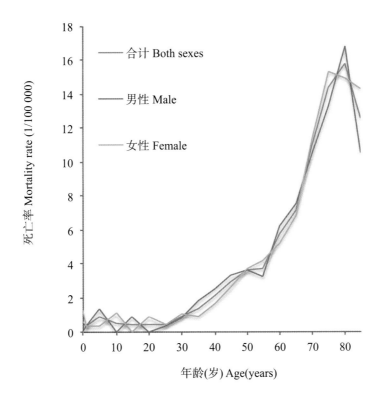

图 5.19.4 2017 年北京市户籍居民脑癌年龄别死亡率
Figure 5.19.4 Age-specific mortality rates of brain cancer in Beijing, 2017

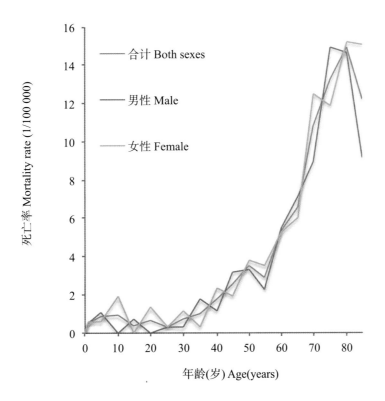

图 5.19.5 2017 年北京市城区户籍居民脑癌年龄别死亡率
Figure 5.19.5 Age-specific mortality rates of brain cancer in urban areas of Beijing, 2017

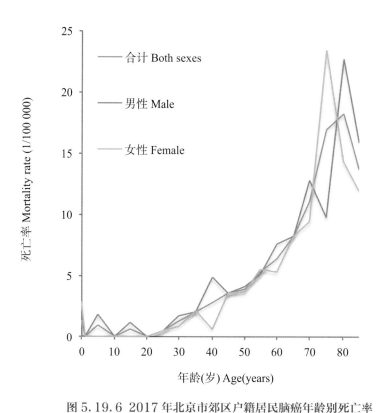

图 5.19.6 2017 年北京市郊区户籍居民脑癌年龄别死亡率

Figure 5.19.6 Age-specific mortality rates of brain cancer in peri-urban areas of Beijing, 2017

全部脑恶性肿瘤（C71）新发病例中，有明确亚部位的病例数占 52.95%。其中额叶是最常见的发病部位，占 25.08%；其后依次为交搭跨越、颞叶和大脑（除外脑叶及脑室），分别占全部脑恶性肿瘤的 21.67%、19.81% 和 9.91%（图 5.19.7）。

About 52.95% cases were assigned to specified categories of brain cancer (C71) sites. Among those, frontal lobe was the most common site, accounting for 25.08% of all cases, followed by the overlapping part (21.67%), temporal lobe (19.81%) and cerebrum (except lobes and ventricles) (9.91%) (Figure 5.19.7).

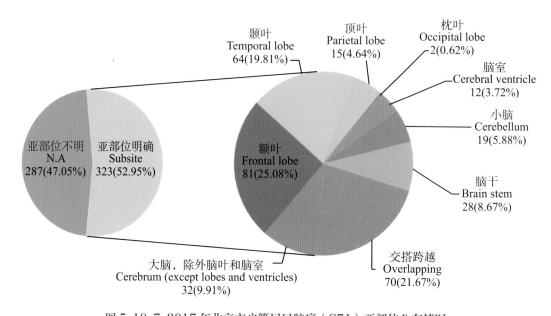

图 5.19.7 2017 年北京市户籍居民脑癌（C71）亚部位分布情况

Figure 5.19.7 Subsite distribution of brain cancer(C71) in Beijing, 2017

（撰稿 李晴雨，校稿 张倩）

5.20 甲状腺（C73）

2017 年，北京市甲状腺癌新发病例数为 4 672 例，占全部恶性肿瘤发病的 9.33%，位居恶性肿瘤发病第 4 位；其中男性 1 209 例，女性 3 463 例，城区 3 074 例，郊区 1 598 例。甲状腺癌粗发病率为 34.33/10 万，中标发病率为 30.76/10 万，世标发病率为 25.75/10 万；女性世标发病率为男性的 2.78 倍，城区世标发病率是郊区的 1.21 倍。0~74 岁累积发病率为 2.29%（表 5.20.1）。

5.20 Thyroid (C73)

There were 4,672 new cases diagnosed as thyroid cancer (1,209 males and 3,463 females, 3,074 in urban areas and 1,598 in peri-urban areas), accounting for 9.33% of all cancers in 2017. Thyroid cancer was the 4th common cancer in Beijing. The crude incidence rate was 34.33 per 100,000, with an ASR China and an ASR World of 30.76 and 25.75 per 100,000, respectively. The ASR World for incidence was 178% higher in females than in males and 21% higher in urban areas than in peri-urban areas. The cumulative incidence rate for subjects aged 0 to 74 years was 2.29% (Table 5.20.1).

表 5.20.1 2017 年北京市户籍居民甲状腺癌发病情况
Table 5.20.1 Incidence of thyroid cancer in Beijing, 2017

地区 Areas	性别 Sex	例数 No. cases	粗率 Crude rate (1/10⁵)	构成比 Freq.（%）	中标率 ASR China (1/10⁵)	世标率 ASR World (1/10⁵)	累积率 Cumulative rate(0~74, %)	顺位 Rank
全市 All areas	合计 Both	4 672	34.33	9.33	30.76	25.75	2.29	4
	男性 Male	1 209	17.80	4.88	16.73	13.66	1.17	8
	女性 Female	3 463	50.79	13.68	44.93	37.95	3.41	3
城区 Urban areas	合计 Both	3 074	36.42	9.32	33.33	27.66	2.46	4
	男性 Male	818	19.43	5.08	18.74	15.19	1.30	8
	女性 Female	2 256	53.33	13.36	48.07	40.25	3.63	3
郊区 Peri-urban areas	合计 Both	1 598	30.91	9.36	26.78	22.84	2.02	4
	男性 Male	391	15.14	4.53	13.64	11.33	0.97	8
	女性 Female	1 207	46.63	14.31	40.07	34.44	3.07	3

2017 年，北京市甲状腺癌死亡病例数为 110 例，占全部恶性肿瘤死亡的 0.42%，位居恶性肿瘤死亡第 22 位；其中男性 39 例，女性 71 例，城区 74 例，郊区 36 例。甲状腺癌死亡率为 0.81/10 万，中标和世标死亡率均为 0.35/10 万；女性世标死亡率为男性的 1.78 倍，城区和郊区世标死亡率差异不明显，分别为 0.36/10 万和 0.35/10 万。0~74 岁累积死亡率为 0.04%（表 5.20.2）。

A total of 110 cases died of thyroid cancer (39 males and 71 females, 74 in urban areas and 36 in peri-urban areas), accounting for 0.42% of all cancer deaths in 2017. Thyroid cancer was the 22nd leading cause of cancer deaths in all cancers. The crude mortality rate was 0.81 per 100,000, with the same ASR China and ASR World of 0.35 per 100,000. The mortality rate of ASR World was 78% higher in females than in males. The disparity of ASR World for the mortality in urban and peri-urban areas was not significant, with 0.36 per 100,000 and 0.35 per 100,000, respectively. The cumulative mortality rate for subjects aged 0 to 74 years was 0.04% (Table 5.20.2).

表 5.20.2 2017 年北京市户籍居民甲状腺癌死亡情况
Table 5.20.2 Mortality of thyroid cancer in Beijing, 2017

地区 Areas	性别 Sex	例数 No. deaths	粗率 Crude rate （1/10^5）	构成比 Freq.（%）	中标率 ASR China （1/10^5）	世标率 ASR World （1/10^5）	累积率 Cumulative rate(0~74, %)	顺位 Rank
全市 All areas	合计 Both	110	0.81	0.42	0.35	0.35	0.04	22
	男性 Male	39	0.57	0.25	0.24	0.25	0.03	19
	女性 Female	71	1.04	0.67	0.45	0.44	0.05	18
城区 Urban areas	合计 Both	74	0.88	0.44	0.35	0.36	0.04	20
	男性 Male	25	0.59	0.25	0.23	0.23	0.03	19
	女性 Female	49	1.16	0.70	0.47	0.47	0.05	18
郊区 Peri-urban areas	合计 Both	36	0.70	0.40	0.34	0.35	0.04	22
	男性 Male	14	0.54	0.25	0.27	0.28	0.02	19
	女性 Female	22	0.85	0.62	0.41	0.41	0.05	19

北京市甲状腺癌世标发病率由 2008 年的 4.07/10 万上升到 2017 年的 25.75/10 万，10 年间发病率年均变化百分比为 26.07%（P<0.001）；男性和女性 10 年间发病率年均变化百分比分别为 28.39%（P<0.001）和 25.30%（P<0.001）。北京市甲状腺癌世标死亡率由 2008 年的 0.43/10 万下降到 2017 年的 0.35/10 万，10 年间死亡率年均变化百分比为 -2.66%（P=0.030）；男性和女性 10 年间死亡率年均变化百分比分别为 -2.07%（P=0.047）和 -3.15%（P=0.110）。

甲状腺癌好发于 25~64 岁人群，甲状腺癌发病率在 0~19 岁人群中较低，自 20 岁起快速增长，在 35~39 岁组达到高峰，随后逐渐下降；除 85 岁及以上年龄组人群外，女性各年龄段发病率均高于男性（图 5.20.1）。甲状腺癌死亡率在 40 岁之前很低，之后各年龄组整体呈现上升趋势，至 85 岁及以上年龄组达到高峰；除 55~59 岁和 85 岁及以上年龄组，其他年龄组女性死亡率均高于男性（图 5.20.4）。城区和郊区年龄别发病率、死亡率变化有一定差别，但总体趋势相同，波动较为明显（图 5.20.2 和图 5.20.3，图 5.20.5 和图 5.20.6）。

The ASR World for incidence of thyroid cancer increased from 4.07 per 100,000 in 2008 to 25.75 per 100,000 in 2017, and the APC of ASR World for incidence was 26.07% (P<0.001). The APCs of ASR World for incidence of thyroid cancer in males and females were 28.39% (P<0.001) and 25.30% (P<0.001), respectively. The ASR World for mortality of thyroid cancer decreased from 0.43 per 100,000 in 2008 to 0.35 per 100,000 in 2017, and the APC of ASR World for mortality was -2.66% (P =0.030). The APCs of ASR World for mortality of thyroid cancer in males and females were -2.07% (P=0.047) and -3.15% (P=0.110), respectively.

The incidence of thyroid cancer was common in the age groups between 25-64 years old. The age-specific incidence rate of thyroid cancer was relatively low at the age group of 0-19 years old, and the rate increased sharply in the older groups, peaking at the age group of 35-39 years old, but started to go down gradually from age 40 onwards. Except for the age group of 85+ years old, the age-specific incidence rates were higher for females than for males in all age groups (Figure 5.20.1). The mortality rate of thyroid cancer was relatively low before 40 years old, but the rate increased with slightly fluctuation in older groups, peaking at the age group of 85+ years old. Except for the age groups of 55~59 years old and 85+ years old, the age-specific mortality rates were higher for females than for males in all age groups (Figure 5.20.4). There were some differences in age-specific incidence and mortality rates in urban and peri-urban areas, but the overall trends were same. The age-specific incidence and mortality rates showed huge fluctuations (Figure 5.20.2-5.20.3, Figure 5.20.5-5.20.6).

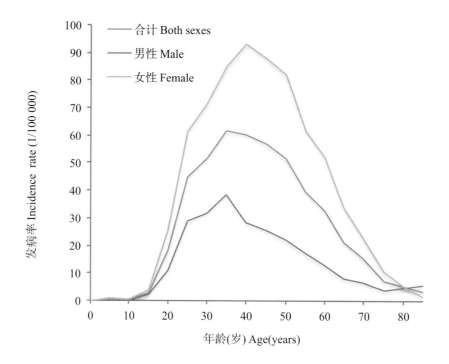

图 5.20.1 2017 年北京市户籍居民甲状腺癌年龄别发病率
Figure 5.20.1 Age-specific incidence rates of thyroid cancer in Beijing, 2017

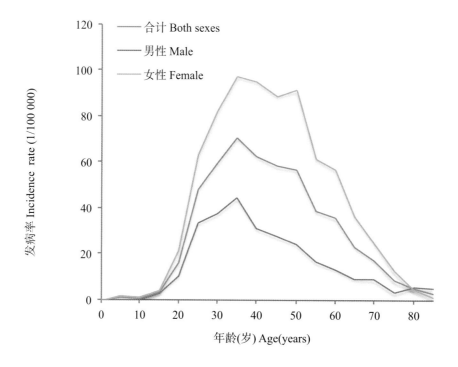

图 5.20.2 2017 年北京市城区户籍居民甲状腺癌年龄别发病率
Figure 5.20.2 Age-specific incidence rates of thyroid cancer in urban areas of Beijing, 2017

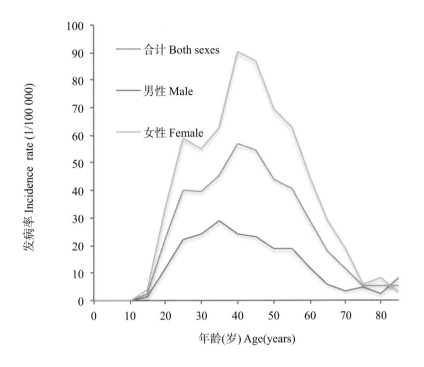

图 5.20.3 2017 年北京市郊区户籍居民甲状腺癌年龄别发病率
Figure 5.20.3 Age-specific incidence rates of thyroid cancer in peri-urban areas of Beijing, 2017

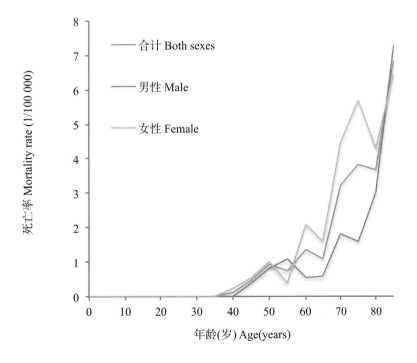

图 5.20.4 2017 年北京市户籍居民甲状腺癌年龄别死亡率
Figure 5.20.4 Age-specific mortality rates of thyroid cancer in Beijing, 2017

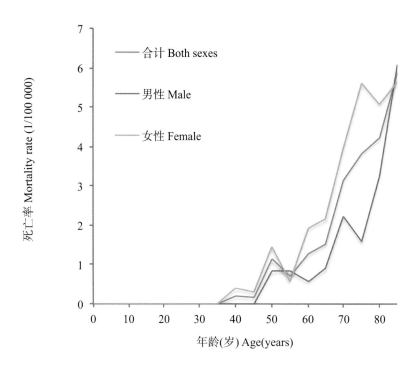

图 5.20.5 2017 年北京市城区户籍居民甲状腺癌年龄别死亡率
Figure 5.20.5 Age-specific mortality rates of thyroid cancer in urban areas of Beijing, 2017

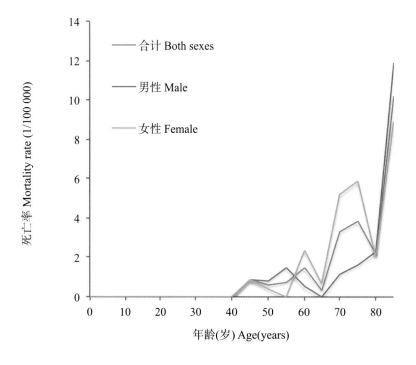

图 5.20.6 2017 年北京市郊区户籍居民甲状腺癌年龄别死亡率
Figure 5.20.6 Age-specific mortality rates of thyroid cancer in peri-urban areas of Beijing, 2017

2017 年，北京市甲状腺癌世标发病率在 16 个辖区间有显著差异，城区发病率高于郊区。甲状腺癌世标死亡率在 16 个辖区间差异不明显（图 5.20.7 和图 5.20.8 ）。

In 2017, there were significant differences between the 16 districts in ASR World for incidence of thyroid cancer in Beijing. The incidence rate was higher in urban areas than in peri-urban areas. There was slight difference between the 16 districts in ASR World for mortality of thyroid cancer in Beijing (Figure 5.20.7-5.20.8).

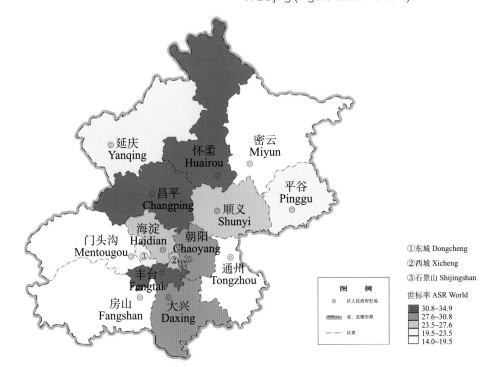

图 5.20.7 2017 年北京市户籍居民甲状腺癌发病率（1/10⁵）地区分布情况
Figure 5.20.7 Incidence rates of thyroid cancer by district in Beijing, 2017（1/10⁵）

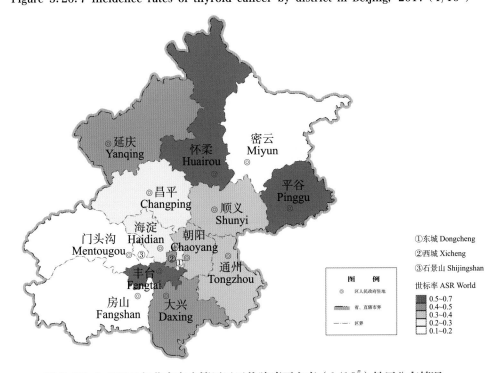

图 5.20.8 2017 年北京市户籍居民甲状腺癌死亡率（1/10⁵）地区分布情况
Figure 5.20.8 Mortality rates of thyroid cancer by district in Beijing, 2017（1/10⁵）

（撰稿　杨雷，校稿　程杨杨）

5.21 淋巴瘤 （C81-85, C88, C90, C96）

2017年，北京市淋巴瘤新发病例数为 1 439 例，占全部恶性肿瘤发病的 2.87%，位居恶性肿瘤发病第 12 位；其中男性 814 例，女性 625 例，城区 983 例，郊区 456 例。淋巴瘤发病率为 10.57/10 万，中标发病率为 5.85/10 万，世标发病率为 5.62/10 万；男性世标发病率为女性的 1.39 倍，城区世标发病率为郊区的 1.18 倍。0~74 岁累积发病率为 0.63%（表 5.21.1）。

5.21 Lymphoma (C81-85, C88, C90, C96)

There were 1,439 new cases diagnosed as lymphoma (814 males and 625 females, 983 in urban areas and 456 in peri-urban areas), accounting for 2.87% of new cases of all cancers in 2017. Lymphoma was the 12th common cancer in Beijing. The crude incidence rate was 10.57 per 100,000, with an ASR China and an ASR World of 5.85 and 5.62 per 100,000, respectively. The ASR World for incidence was 39% higher in males than in females and 18% higher in urban areas than in peri-urban areas. The cumulative incidence rate for subjects aged 0 to 74 years was 0.63% (Table 5.21.1).

表 5.21.1 2017 年北京市户籍居民淋巴瘤发病情况
Table 5.21.1 Incidence of lymphoma in Beijing, 2017

地区 Areas	性别 Sex	例数 No. cases	粗率 Crude rate （1/10^5）	构成比 Freq.（%）	中标率 ASR China （1/10^5）	世标率 ASR World （1/10^5）	累积率 Cumulative rate(0~74, %)	顺位 Rank
全市 All areas	合计 Both	1 439	10.57	2.87	5.85	5.62	0.63	12
	男性 Male	814	11.99	3.29	6.82	6.56	0.73	10
	女性 Female	625	9.17	2.47	4.92	4.72	0.52	11
城区 Urban areas	合计 Both	983	11.65	2.98	6.21	5.95	0.67	12
	男性 Male	530	12.59	3.29	6.87	6.61	0.74	10
	女性 Female	453	10.71	2.68	5.58	5.32	0.61	9
郊区 Peri-urban areas	合计 Both	456	8.82	2.67	5.23	5.05	0.55	15
	男性 Male	284	11.00	3.29	6.72	6.48	0.72	10
	女性 Female	172	6.65	2.04	3.82	3.71	0.39	13

2017 年，北京市淋巴瘤死亡病例数为 929 例，占全部恶性肿瘤死亡的 3.57%，位居恶性肿瘤死亡第 10 位；其中男性 522 例，女性 407 例，城区 618 例，郊区 311 例。淋巴瘤死亡率为 6.83/10 万，中标死亡率为 2.99/10 万，世标死亡率为 2.93/10 万；男性世标死亡率为女性的 1.36 倍，郊区世标死亡率为城区的 1.05 倍。0~74 岁累积死亡率为 0.33%（表 5.21.2）。

A total of 929 cases died of lymphoma (522 males and 407 females, 618 in urban areas and 311 in peri-urban areas), accounting for 3.57% of all cancer deaths in 2017. Lymphoma was the 10th leading causes of cancer deaths in all cancers. The crude mortality rate was 6.83 per 100,000, with an ASR China and an ASR World of 2.99 and 2.93 per 100,000, respectively. The ASR World for mortality was 36% higher in males than in females and 5% higher in peri-urban areas than in urban areas. The cumulative mortality rate for subjects aged 0 to 74 years was 0.33% (Table 5.21.2).

表 5.21.2 2017 年北京市户籍居民淋巴瘤死亡情况
Table 5.21.2 Mortality of lymphoma in Beijing, 2017

地区 Areas	性别 Sex	例数 No. deaths	粗率 Crude rate （1/10⁵）	构成比 Freq.（%）	中标率 ASR China （1/10⁵）	世标率 ASR World （1/10⁵）	累积率 Cumulative rate(0~74, %)	顺位 Rank
全市 All areas	合计 Both	929	6.83	3.57	2.99	2.93	0.33	10
	男性 Male	522	7.69	3.37	3.49	3.39	0.38	10
	女性 Female	407	5.97	3.86	2.53	2.50	0.28	8
城区 Urban areas	合计 Both	618	7.32	3.64	2.94	2.87	0.32	9
	男性 Male	341	8.10	3.42	3.33	3.24	0.36	9
	女性 Female	277	6.55	3.95	2.59	2.53	0.29	8
郊区 Peri-urban areas	合计 Both	311	6.02	3.43	3.07	3.02	0.33	10
	男性 Male	181	7.01	3.28	3.77	3.66	0.41	9
	女性 Female	130	5.02	3.67	2.42	2.43	0.27	9

北京市淋巴瘤世标发病率由 2008 年的 5.27/10 万上升到 2017 年的 5.62/10 万，年均变化百分比为 0.57%（P=0.321）；男性和女性发病 10 年间年

The ASR World for incidence of lymphoma increased from 5.27 per 100,000 in 2008 to 5.62 per 100,000 in 2017; the APC of ASR World for incidence was 0.57% (P=0.321). The APCs of ASR World for incidence of

均变化百分比分别为 0.96%（*P*=0.084）和 0.05%（*P*=0.946）。北京市淋巴瘤世标死亡率由 2008 年的 2.63/10 万上升到 2017 年的 2.93/10 万，年均变化百分比为 1.00%（*P*=0.082）；男性和女性死亡 10 年间年均变化百分比分别为 0.54%（*P*=0.397）和 1.63%（*P*=0.037）。

　　淋巴瘤年龄别发病率和死亡率在 40 岁以前处于较低水平，自 40 岁以后快速上升，发病率在 75~79 岁年龄组达到高峰，死亡率在 85 岁及以上年龄组达到高峰（图 5.21.1 至图 5.21.6）。45 岁及以上各年龄组男性发病率和死亡率均高于女性（图 5.21.1 和图 5.21.4）。城区和郊区年龄别发病率、死亡率变化总体趋势类似，但郊区发病率和死亡率波动更明显（图 5.21.2 和 5.21.3，图 5.21.5 和 5.21.6）。

lymphoma in males and females were 0.96% (*P*=0.084) and 0.05% (*P*=0.946), respectively. The ASR World for mortality of lymphoma increased from 2.63 per 100,000 in 2008 to 2.93 per 100,000 in 2017; the APC of ASR World for mortality was 1.00% (*P*=0.082). The APCs of ASR World for mortality of lymphoma in males and females were 0.54% (*P*=0.397) and 1.63% (*P*=0.037), respectively.

The age-specific incidence and mortality rates of lymphoma were relatively low in people below 40 years old, and the rates increased sharply in people older than that (Figure 5.21.1- 5.21.6). The age-specific incidence reached the peak at the age group of 75~79 years; the age-specific mortality reached the peak at the age group of 85 years and above. Rates in males were higher than those in females at the age groups of 45+ years (Figure 5.21.1, Figure 5.21.4). The overall trends of age-specific incidence and mortality rates between urban and peri-urban areas were same, but in peri-urban areas showed huge fluctuation (Figure 5.21.2-5.21.3, Figure 5.21.5-5.21.6).

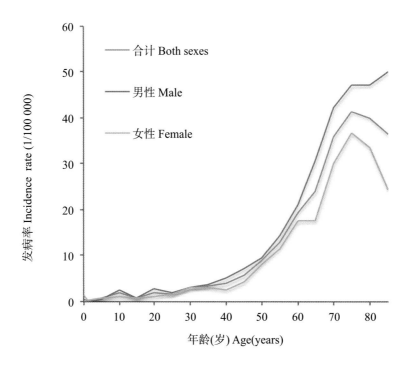

图 5.21.1 2017 年北京市户籍居民淋巴瘤年龄别发病率
Figure 5.21.1 Age-specific incidence rates of lymphoma in Beijing, 2017

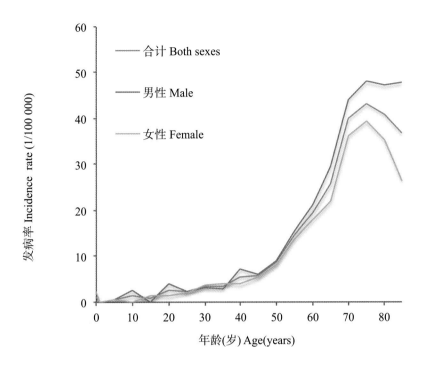

图 5.21.2 2017 年北京市城区户籍居民淋巴瘤年龄别发病率
Figure 5.21.2 Age-specific incidence rates of lymphoma in urban areas of Beijing, 2017

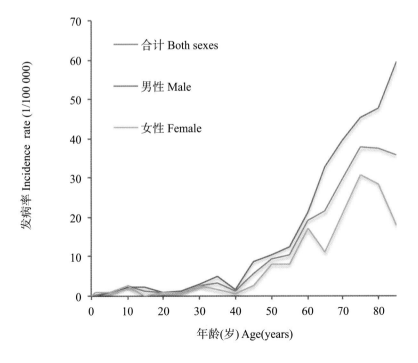

图 5.21.3 2017 年北京市郊区户籍居民淋巴瘤年龄别发病率
Figure 5.21.3 Age-specific incidence rates of lymphoma in peri-urban areas of Beijing, 2017

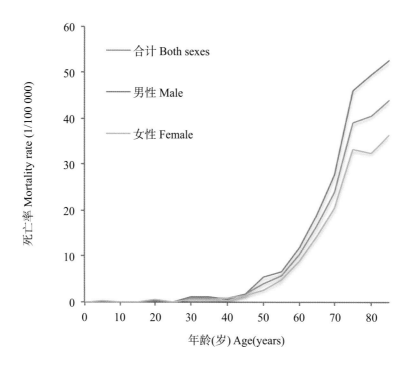

图 5.21.4 2017 年北京市户籍居民淋巴瘤年龄别死亡率
Figure 5.21.4 Age-specific mortality rates of lymphoma in Beijing, 2017

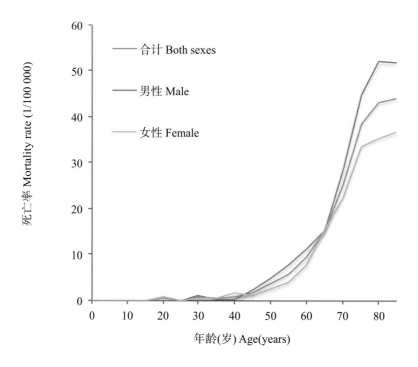

图 5.21.5 2017 年北京市城区户籍居民淋巴瘤年龄别死亡率
Figure 5.21.5 Age-specific mortality rates of lymphoma in urban areas of Beijing, 2017

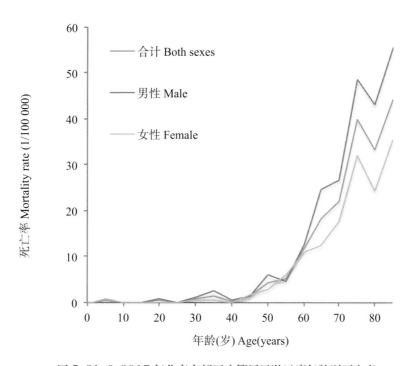

图 5.21.6 2017 年北京市郊区户籍居民淋巴瘤年龄别死亡率

Figure 5.21.6 Age-specific mortality rates of lymphoma in peri-urban areas of Beijing, 2017

2017 年，北京市淋巴瘤世标发病率在 16 个辖区间有显著差异，城区发病率高于郊区。世标死亡率在 16 个辖区间差异不明显（图 5.21.7 和图 5.21.8）。

In 2017, there were significant differences between the 16 districts in ASR World for incidence of lymphoma in Beijing. The incidence rate was higher in urban areas than in peri-urban areas. There was slight difference between the 16 districts in ASR World for mortality of lymphoma cancer in Beijing (Figure 5.21.7-5.21.8).

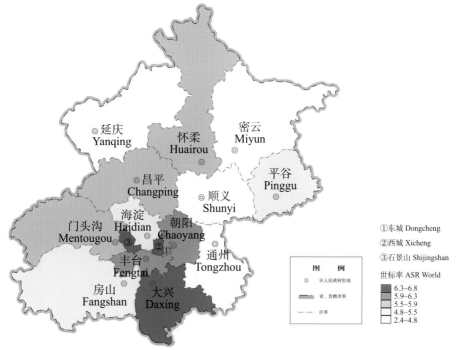

图 5.21.7 2017 年北京市户籍居民淋巴瘤发病率（1/10^5）地区分布情况

Figure 5.21.7 Incidence rates of lymphoma by district in Beijing, 2017 (1/10^5)

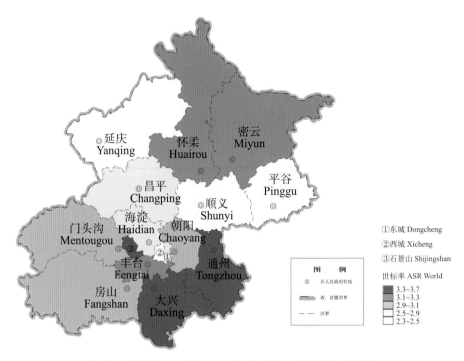

图 5.21.8 2017 年北京市户籍居民淋巴瘤死亡率（1/10^5）地区分布情况
Figure 5.21.8 Mortality rates of lymphoma by district in Beijing, 2017 (1/10^5)

全部淋巴瘤病例中有明确病理分型的占 99.17%。其中非霍奇金淋巴瘤的其他和未特指类型是最主要的病理类型，占 37.60%；其后依次为多发性骨髓瘤和恶性浆细胞肿瘤（24.60%）、弥漫性非霍奇金淋巴瘤（20.99%）、滤泡性非霍奇金淋巴瘤（6.53%）、霍奇金淋巴瘤（4.59%）、周围和皮肤 T 细胞淋巴瘤（3.89%）和恶性免疫增生性疾病（0.97%）。其他和未特指的淋巴、造血和有关组织的恶性肿瘤占 0.83%（图 5.21.9）。

Among all lymphoma cases, 99.17% had morphological verification. Among them, other and unspecified types of non-Hodgkin's lymphoma was the most common histological type, accounting for 37.60% of all cases, followed by the multiple myeloma and the malignant plasma cell neoplasms (24.60%), the diffuse non-Hodgkin's lymphoma (20.99%), the follicular non-Hodgkin's lymphoma (6.53%), the Hodgkin's disease (4.59%), the peripheral and cutaneous T-cell lymphoma (3.89%), the malignant immunoproliferative disease (0.97%), and the other and unspecified lymphoma (0.83%) (Figure 5.21.9).

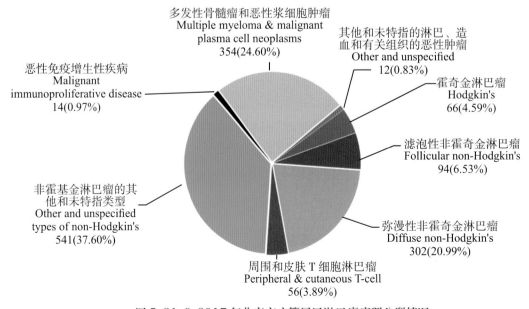

图 5.21.9 2017 年北京市户籍居民淋巴瘤病理分型情况
Figure 5.21.9 Morphological distribution of lymphoma in Beijing, 2017

（撰稿 程杨杨，校稿 张希）

5.22 白血病（C91-95, D45-47）

5.22 Leukemia (C91-95, D45-47)

　　2017年,北京市白血病新发病例数为1 217例,占全部恶性肿瘤发病的2.43%，位居恶性肿瘤发病第15位；其中男性697例，女性520例，城区760例, 郊区457例。白血病发病率为8.94/10万,中标发病率为5.69/10万, 世标发病率为5.93/10万；男性世标发病率为女性的1.33倍，郊区世标发病率为城区的1.06倍。0~74岁累积发病率为0.55%（表5.22.1）。

　　There were 1,217 new cases diagnosed as leukemia (697 males and 520 females, 760 in urban areas and 457 in peri-urban areas), accounting for 2.43% of new cases of all cancers in 2017. Leukemia was the 15th common cancer in Beijing. The crude incidence rate was 8.94 per 100,000, with an ASR China and an ASR World of 5.69 and 5.93 per 100,000, respectively. The ASR World for incidence was 33% higher in males than in females and 6% higher in peri-urban areas than in urban areas. The cumulative incidence rate for subjects aged 0 to 74 years was 0.55% (Table 5.22.1).

表 5.22.1　2017 年北京市户籍居民白血病发病情况
Table 5.22.1 Incidence of leukemia in Beijing, 2017

地区 Areas	性别 Sex	例数 No. cases	粗率 Crude rate (1/10⁵)	构成比 Freq.（%）	中标率 ASR China (1/10⁵)	世标率 ASR World (1/10⁵)	累积率 Cumulative rate(0~74, %)	顺位 Rank
全市 All areas	合计 Both	1 217	8.94	2.43	5.69	5.93	0.55	15
	男性 Male	697	10.26	2.82	6.49	6.78	0.61	12
	女性 Female	520	7.63	2.05	4.93	5.10	0.48	13
城区 Urban areas	合计 Both	760	9.00	2.30	5.56	5.80	0.53	15
	男性 Male	452	10.74	2.81	6.44	6.78	0.61	12
	女性 Female	308	7.28	1.82	4.74	4.86	0.46	15
郊区 Peri-urban areas	合计 Both	457	8.84	2.68	5.93	6.15	0.57	14
	男性 Male	245	9.49	2.84	6.56	6.78	0.62	12
	女性 Female	212	8.19	2.51	5.33	5.54	0.52	11

2017 年，北京市白血病死亡病例数为 867 例，占全部恶性肿瘤死亡的 3.33%，位居恶性肿瘤死亡第 11 位；其中男性 527 例，女性 340 例，城区 567 例，郊区 300 例。白血病死亡率为 6.37/10 万，中标死亡率为 3.29/10 万，世标死亡率为 3.24/10 万；男性世标死亡率为女性的 1.54 倍，郊区世标死亡率为城区的 1.06 倍。0~74 岁累积死亡率为 0.32%（表 5.22.2）。

A total of 867 cases died of leukemia (527 males and 340 females, 567 in urban areas and 300 in peri-urban areas), accounting for 3.33% of all cancer deaths in 2017. Leukemia was the 11th leading cause of cancer deaths in all cancers. The crude mortality rate was 6.37 per 100,000, with an ASR China and an ASR World of 3.29 and 3.24 per 100,000, respectively. The ASR World for mortality was 54% higher in males than in females and 6% higher in peri-urban areas than in urban areas. The cumulative mortality rate for subjects aged 0 to 74 years was 0.32% (Table 5.22.2).

表 5.22.2　2017 年北京市户籍居民白血病死亡情况
Table 5.22.2 Mortality of leukemia in Beijing, 2017

地区 Areas	性别 Sex	例数 No. deaths	粗率 Crude rate （1/10⁵）	构成比 Freq.（%）	中标率 ASR China （1/10⁵）	世标率 ASR World （1/10⁵）	累积率 Cumulative rate(0~74, %)	顺位 Rank
全市 All areas	合计 Both	867	6.37	3.33	3.29	3.24	0.32	11
	男性 Male	527	7.76	3.40	4.04	3.96	0.39	8
	女性 Female	340	4.99	3.22	2.60	2.58	0.26	10
城区 Urban areas	合计 Both	567	6.72	3.34	3.15	3.16	0.32	11
	男性 Male	338	8.03	3.39	3.64	3.63	0.37	10
	女性 Female	229	5.41	3.27	2.74	2.75	0.27	11
郊区 Peri-urban areas	合计 Both	300	5.80	3.31	3.50	3.36	0.33	12
	男性 Male	189	7.32	3.43	4.65	4.43	0.42	8
	女性 Female	111	4.29	3.13	2.38	2.31	0.24	10

北京市白血病世标发病率由 2008 年的 5.41/10 万上升到 2017 年[6] 的 5.93/10 万，年均变化百分比为 -0.53%（P=0.589）；男性和

The ASR World for incidence of leukemia increased from 5.41 per 100,000 in 2008 to 5.93 per 100,000 in 2017; the APC of ASR World for incidence was -0.53%(P=0.589). The APCs of ASR World

---

6. 2008—2016 年白血病统计范围为 ICD-10 编码 C91-95，2017 年统计范围为 C91-95 和 D45-47。

Codes C91-95 in the ICD-10 were included in the analysis as leukemia from 2008 to 2016. Codes C91-95 and D45-47 were included in the analysis as leukemia in 2017.

女性发病 10 年间年均变化百分比分别为 -0.26%（P=0.775）和 -0.96%（P=0.458）。北京市白血病世标死亡率由 2008 年的 2.97/10 万上升到 2017 年的 3.24/10 万，年均变化百分比为 -1.91%（P=0.100）；男性和女性死亡 10 年间年均变化百分比分别为 -1.12%（P=0.345）和 -3.00%（P=0.030）。

白血病年龄别发病率在 0~4 岁组较高，在 5 岁后趋于平缓，40~44 岁开始快速升高，在 80~84 岁达到高峰（图 5.22.1 至图 5.22.3）。白血病年龄别死亡率在 0 岁组较高，在 1 岁后趋于平缓，50~54 岁开始快速升高，在 85 岁及以上年龄组达到高峰（图 5.22.4 至图 5.22.6）。45 岁后，男性发病率和死亡率均显著高于女性（图 5.22.1 和图 5.22.4）。城区和郊区年龄别发病率和死亡率总体变化趋势类似，但 70 岁以后波动水平有一定差异（图 5.22.2 和图 5.22.3，图 5.22.5 和图 5.22.6）。

for incidence of leukemia in males and females were -0.26% (P=0.775) and -0.96% (P=0.458), respectively. The ASR World for mortality of leukemia increased from 2.97 per 100,000 in 2008 to 3.24 per 100,000 in 2017. The APC of ASR world for mortality was -1.91%(P=0.100). The APCs of ASR World for mortality of leukemia in males and females were -1.12% (P=0.345) and -3.00% (P=0.030), respectively.

The age-specific incidence rate was relatively high at the age group of 0~4 years, and remained relatively stable since 5 years old. It dramatically increased at the age group of 40~44 years, and peaked at the age of 80~84 years(Figure 5.22.1-5.22.3). The age-specific mortality rate was relatively high at the age group of 0 years, and remained relatively stable since 1 year old. It dramatically increased at the age group of 50~54 years, and peaked at the age group of 85 years and above (Figure 5.22.4-5.22.6). The incidence and mortality rates in males were significantly higher than those in females after 45 years old (Figure 5.22.1, Figure 5.22.4). The general trends of age-specific incidence and mortality in urban and peri-urban areas were similar, but there were certain differences in the fluctuation levels at the age groups of 70+ years (Figure 5.22.2-5.22.3, Figure 5.22.5-5.22.6).

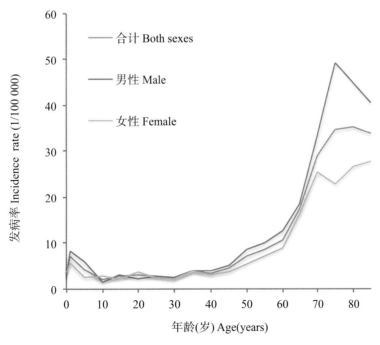

图 5.22.1 2017 年北京市户籍居民白血病年龄别发病率
Figure 5.22.1 Age-specific incidence rates of leukemia in Beijing, 2017

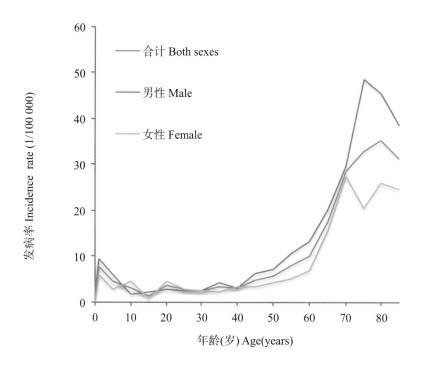

图 5.22.2 2017 年北京市城区户籍居民白血病年龄别发病率
Figure 5.22.2 Age-specific incidence rates of leukemia in urban areas of Beijing, 2017

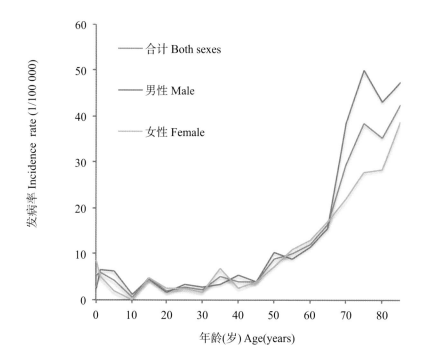

图 5.22.3 2017 年北京市郊区户籍居民白血病年龄别发病率
Figure 5.22.3 Age-specific incidence rates of leukemia in peri-urban areas of Beijing, 2017

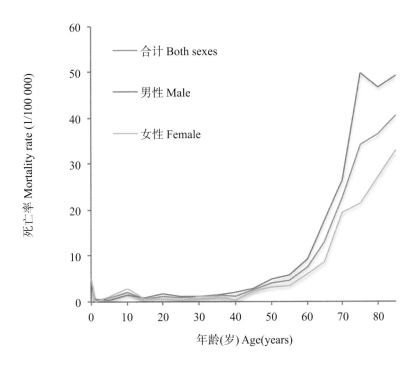

图 5.22.4 2017 年北京市户籍居民白血病年龄别死亡率
Figure 5.22.4 Age-specific mortality rates of leukemia in Beijing, 2017

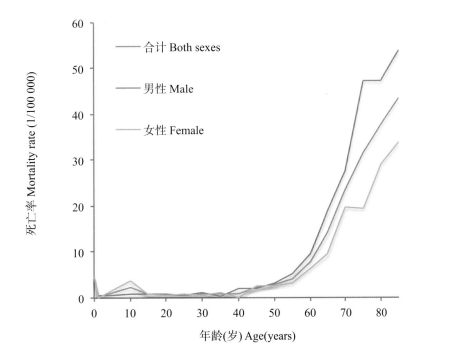

图 5.22.5 2017 年北京市城区户籍居民白血病年龄别死亡率
Figure 5.22.5 Age-specific mortality rates of leukemia in urban areas of Beijing, 2017

（撰稿　程杨杨，校稿　张希）

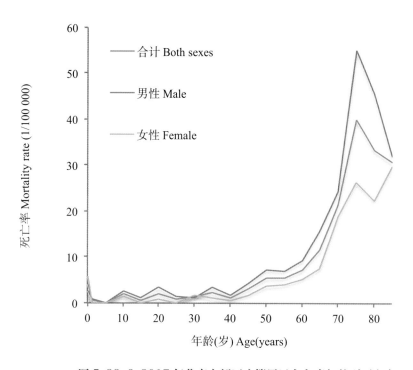

图 5.22.6　2017 年北京市郊区户籍居民白血病年龄别死亡率
Figure 5.22.6 Age-specific mortality rates of leukemia in peri-urban areas of Beijing, 2017

白血病（C91-95）新发病例（794 例）中，最主要的病理类型是髓样白血病，占 51.89%；其后依次为淋巴样白血病（22.29%）和单核细胞白血病（4.03%）（图 5.22.7）。

Among the new cases of leukemia, myeloid leukemia was the most common histological type, accounting for 51.89%, followed by lymphoid leukemia (22.29%) and monocytic leukemia (4.03%) (Figure 5.22.7).

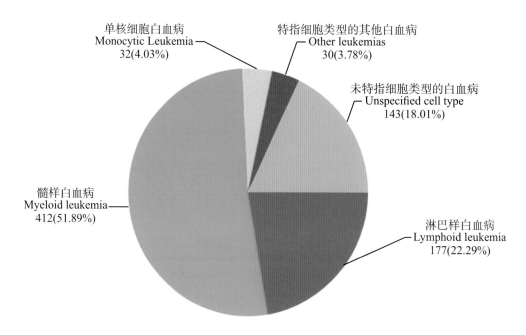

图 5.22.7　2017 年北京市户籍居民白血病（C91-95）病理分型情况
Figure 5.22.7 Morphological distribution of leukemia (C91-95) in Beijing, 2017

5.23 皮肤恶性黑色素瘤（C43）[7]

5.23 Cutaneous malignant melanoma (C43)

2017 年，北京市皮肤恶性黑色素瘤新发病例数为 79 例，占全部恶性肿瘤发病的 0.16%，位居恶性肿瘤发病第 24 位；其中男性 36 例，女性 43 例，城区 56 例，郊区 23 例。皮肤恶性黑色素瘤发病率为 0.58/10 万，中标发病率为 0.34/10 万，世标发病率为 0.31/10 万；女性世标发病率为男性的 1.38 倍，城区世标发病率为郊区的 1.64 倍。0~74 岁累积发病率为 0.03%（表 5.23.1）。

There were 79 new cases diagnosed as cutaneous malignant melanoma (36 males and 43 females, 56 in urban areas and 23 in peri-urban areas), accounting for 0.16% of new cases of all cancers in 2017. Cutaneous malignant melanoma was the 24th common cancer in Beijing. The crude incidence rate was 0.58 per 100,000, with an ASR China and an ASR World of 0.34 and 0.31 per 100,000, respectively. The ASR World for incidence was 38% higher in females than in males and 64% higher in urban areas than in peri-urban areas. The cumulative incidence rate for subjects aged 0 to 74 years was 0.03% (Table 5.23.1).

表 5.23.1 2017 年北京市户籍居民皮肤恶性黑色素瘤发病情况
Table 5.23.1 Incidence of cutaneous malignant melanoma in Beijing, 2017

地区 Areas	性别 Sex	例数 No. cases	粗率 Crude rate ($1/10^5$)	构成比 Freq.（%）	中标率 ASR China ($1/10^5$)	世标率 ASR World ($1/10^5$)	累积率 Cumulative rate(0~74, %)	顺位 Rank
全市 All areas	合计 Both	79	0.58	0.16	0.34	0.31	0.03	24
	男性 Male	36	0.53	0.15	0.29	0.26	0.03	21
	女性 Female	43	0.63	0.17	0.38	0.36	0.04	21
城区 Urban areas	合计 Both	56	0.66	0.17	0.40	0.37	0.04	24
	男性 Male	24	0.57	0.15	0.29	0.26	0.03	21
	女性 Female	32	0.76	0.19	0.51	0.48	0.05	21
郊区 Peri-urban areas	合计 Both	23	0.44	0.13	0.24	0.23	0.02	24
	男性 Male	12	0.46	0.14	0.29	0.27	0.03	20
	女性 Female	11	0.43	0.13	0.19	0.19	0.02	21

---

7. 因北京市皮肤恶性黑色素瘤发病和死亡例数较少，本章节不包含年龄别发病率和死亡率的统计数据和图表。

Because of few cutaneous malignant melanoma cases and deaths occured in Beijing in 2017, this section does not contain statistical data and charts on age-specific incidence and mortality rates.

2017 年，北京市皮肤恶性黑色素瘤死亡病例数为 58 例，占全部恶性肿瘤死亡的 0.22%，位居恶性肿瘤死亡第 29 位；其中男性 32 例，女性 26 例，城区 38 例，郊区 20 例。死亡率为 0.43/10 万，中标死亡率为 0.21/10 万，世标死亡率为 0.20/10 万；男性世标死亡率为女性的 1.20 倍，郊区世标死亡率是城区的 1.03 倍。0~74 岁累积死亡率为 0.02%（表 5.23.2）。

A total of 58 cases died of cutaneous malignant melanoma (32 males and 26 females, 38 in urban areas and 20 in peri-urban areas), accounting for 0.22% of all cancer deaths in 2017. Cutaneous malignant melanoma was the 29th leading cause of cancer deaths in all cancers. The crude mortality rate was 0.43 per 100,000, with an ASR China and an ASR World of 0.21 and 0.20 per 100,000, respectively. The ASR World for mortality was 20% higher in males than in females and 3% higher in peri-urban areas than in urban areas. The cumulative mortality rate for subjects aged 0 to 74 years was 0.02% (Table 5.23.2).

表 5.23.2 2017 年北京市户籍居民皮肤恶性黑色素瘤死亡情况
Table 5.23.2 Mortality of cutaneous malignant melanoma in Beijing, 2017

地区 Areas	性别 Sex	例数 No. deaths	粗率 Crude rate （1/10⁵）	构成比 Freq.（%）	中标率 ASR China （1/10⁵）	世标率 ASR World （1/10⁵）	累积率 Cumulative rate（0~74, %）	顺位 Rank
全市 All areas	合计 Both	58	0.43	0.22	0.21	0.20	0.02	29
	男性 Male	32	0.47	0.21	0.22	0.22	0.02	25
	女性 Female	26	0.38	0.25	0.20	0.18	0.02	26
城区 Urban areas	合计 Both	38	0.45	0.22	0.20	0.19	0.02	29
	男性 Male	21	0.50	0.21	0.20	0.20	0.01	25
	女性 Female	17	0.40	0.24	0.20	0.19	0.02	26
郊区 Peri-urban areas	合计 Both	20	0.39	0.22	0.21	0.20	0.03	29
	男性 Male	11	0.43	0.20	0.23	0.23	0.04	25
	女性 Female	9	0.35	0.25	0.19	0.17	0.02	26

北京市皮肤恶性黑色素瘤世标发病率由 2008 年的 0.37/10 万下降到 2017 年的 0.31/10 万，年均变化百分比为 −2.22%（P=0.287）；男性和女性发病 10 年间年均变化百分比分别为 −5.04%（P=0.088）和 0.31%（P=0.875）。北京市皮肤恶性黑色素瘤世标死亡率由 2008 年的 0.18/10 万上升到 2017 年的 0.20/10 万，年均变化百分比为 0.35%（P=0.761）；男性和女性死亡 10 年间年均变化百分比分别为 −0.38%（P=0.823）和 1.21%（P=0.595）。

The ASR World for incidence of cutaneous malignant melanoma decreased from 0.37 per 100,000 in 2008 to 0.31 per 100,000 in 2017; the APC of ASR World for incidence was −2.22% (P=0.287). The APCs of ASR World for incidence of cutaneous malignant melanoma in males and females were −5.04% (P=0.088) and 0.31% (P=0.875), respectively. The ASR World for mortality of cutaneous malignant melanoma increased from 0.18 per 100,000 in 2008 to 0.20 per 100,000 in 2017; the APC of ASR World for mortality was 0.35% (P=0.761). The APCs of ASR World for mortality of cutaneous malignant melanoma in males and females were −0.38% (P=0.823) and 1.21% (P=0.595), respectively.

（撰稿　程杨杨，校稿　张希）

附　录
Appendix

附表 1　2017 年北京市户籍居民恶性肿瘤发病主要指标
Appendix table 1　Incidence of all cancers in Beijing, 2017

部位 Sites	男性 Male					
	例数 No.cases	粗率 Crude rate （1/10⁵）	构成比 Freq.（%）	中标率 ASR China （1/10⁵）	世标率 ASR World （1/10⁵）	累积率 Cumulative rate(0~74,%)
口腔 Oral cavity & pharynx	388	5.71	1.57	2.99	3.01	0.35
鼻咽 Nasopharynx	56	0.82	0.23	0.56	0.51	0.06
食管 Esophagus	964	14.19	3.89	6.47	6.61	0.80
胃 Stomach	1 667	24.55	6.73	11.65	11.52	1.37
结直肠 Colon-rectum	3 620	53.30	14.63	25.74	25.55	3.10
肝脏 Liver	1 670	24.59	6.75	12.55	12.54	1.43
胆囊 Gallbladder etc.	572	8.42	2.31	3.83	3.80	0.45
胰腺 Pancreas	811	11.94	3.28	5.77	5.68	0.71
喉 Larynx	274	4.03	1.11	1.99	2.03	0.25
肺 Lung	6 041	88.95	24.41	41.67	41.60	5.18
其他胸腔器官 Other thoracic organs	92	1.35	0.37	0.83	0.81	0.09
骨 Bone	103	1.52	0.42	1.34	1.29	0.10
皮肤黑色素瘤 Melanoma of skin	36	0.53	0.15	0.29	0.26	0.03
乳腺 Breast	31	0.46	0.13	0.22	0.21	0.02
子宫颈 Cervix	—	—	—	—	—	—
子宫体 Uterus	—	—	—	—	—	—
卵巢 Ovary	—	—	—	—	—	—
前列腺 Prostate	1 606	23.65	6.49	10.50	10.30	1.31
睾丸 Testis	39	0.57	0.16	0.58	0.53	0.04
肾 Kidney	1 272	18.73	5.14	10.32	10.03	1.20
膀胱 Bladder	1 257	18.51	5.08	8.51	8.44	0.99
脑 Brain	346	5.09	1.40	3.76	3.63	0.34
甲状腺 Thyroid	1 209	17.80	4.88	16.73	13.66	1.17
淋巴瘤 Lymphoma	814	11.99	3.29	6.82	6.56	0.73
白血病 Leukemia	697	10.26	2.82	6.49	6.78	0.61
其他 Other	1 187	17.49	4.76	9.33	9.57	0.98
所有部位合计 All sites	24 752	364.46	100.00	188.94	184.92	21.31
所有部位除外皮肤 All sites exc.C44	24 511	360.91	99.75	187.18	183.21	21.12

	女性 Female					ICD10
例数 No.cases	粗率 Crude rate （1/10⁵）	构成比 Freq.（%）	中标率 ASR China （1/10⁵）	世标率 ASR World （1/10⁵）	累积率 Cumulative rate （0~74，%）	
231	3.39	0.91	1.81	1.69	0.19	C00-10, C12-14
24	0.35	0.09	0.16	0.16	0.02	C11
219	3.21	0.86	1.11	1.10	0.10	C15
804	11.79	3.18	5.62	5.37	0.58	C16
2 634	38.63	10.40	17.28	16.91	1.96	C18-21
694	10.18	2.74	4.32	4.31	0.46	C22
513	7.52	2.03	3.08	3.01	0.35	C23-24
601	8.81	2.37	3.57	3.52	0.39	C25
17	0.25	0.07	0.09	0.09	0.01	C32
4 084	59.89	16.13	27.38	26.95	3.13	C33-34
55	0.81	0.22	0.42	0.44	0.04	C37-38
61	0.89	0.24	0.63	0.60	0.06	C40-41
43	0.63	0.17	0.38	0.36	0.04	C43
5 119	75.07	20.22	46.27	43.45	4.79	C50
652	9.56	2.58	6.92	6.17	0.61	C53
1 358	19.92	5.36	11.77	11.43	1.31	C54-55
842	12.35	3.33	7.57	7.26	0.79	C56
—	—	—	—	—	—	C61
—	—	—	—	—	—	C62
820	12.03	3.24	5.80	5.74	0.66	C64-66, C68
470	6.89	1.86	2.96	2.92	0.35	C67
320	4.69	1.26	3.07	3.06	0.27	C70-C72
3 463	50.79	13.68	44.93	37.95	3.41	C73
625	9.17	2.47	4.92	4.72	0.52	C81-85, C88, C90, C96
520	7.63	2.05	4.93	5.10	0.48	C91-95, D45-47
1 149	16.85	4.54	9.11	9.01	0.93	Other
25 318	371.30	100.00	214.10	201.32	21.45	All
25 081	367.82	99.06	212.35	199.64	21.26	All sites exc.C44

附表 2 2017 年北京市户籍居民恶性肿瘤死亡主要指标
Appendix table 2 Mortality of all cancers in Beijing, 2017

部位 Sites	男性 Male					
	例数 No.cases	粗率 Crude rate （1/10⁵）	构成比 Freq.（%）	中标率 ASR China （1/10⁵）	世标率 ASR World （1/10⁵）	累积率 Cumulative rate(0~74,%)
口腔 Oral cavity & pharynx	225	3.31	1.45	1.57	1.60	0.19
鼻咽 Nasopharynx	68	1.00	0.44	0.65	0.62	0.06
食管 Esophagus	856	12.60	5.52	5.48	5.57	0.65
胃 Stomach	1 163	17.12	7.50	7.29	7.14	0.75
结直肠 Colon-rectum	1 692	24.91	10.92	10.28	10.19	1.04
肝脏 Liver	1 614	23.77	10.41	11.63	11.60	1.31
胆囊 Gallbladder etc.	452	6.66	2.92	2.82	2.80	0.31
胰腺 Pancreas	766	11.28	4.94	5.27	5.18	0.66
喉 Larynx	113	1.66	0.73	0.70	0.70	0.08
肺 Lung	4 850	71.41	31.29	30.99	30.89	3.63
其他胸腔器官 Other thoracic organs	70	1.03	0.45	0.55	0.52	0.07
骨 Bone	64	0.94	0.41	0.62	0.60	0.05
皮肤黑色素瘤 Melanoma of skin	32	0.47	0.21	0.22	0.22	0.02
乳腺 Breast	10	0.15	0.06	0.06	0.06	0.01
子宫颈 Cervix	—	—	—	—	—	—
子宫体 Uterus	—	—	—	—	—	—
卵巢 Ovary	—	—	—	—	—	—
前列腺 Prostate	613	9.03	3.95	3.06	3.03	0.22
睾丸 Testis	7	0.10	0.05	0.07	0.06	0.00
肾 Kidney	443	6.52	2.86	2.77	2.80	0.29
膀胱 Bladder	524	7.72	3.38	2.64	2.69	0.21
脑 Brain	243	3.58	1.57	2.13	2.06	0.21
甲状腺 Thyroid	39	0.57	0.25	0.24	0.25	0.03
淋巴瘤 Lymphoma	522	7.69	3.37	3.49	3.39	0.38
白血病 Leukemia	527	7.76	3.40	4.04	3.96	0.39
其他 Other	607	8.95	3.92	3.96	4.00	0.42
所有部位合计 **All sites**	15 500	228.23	100.00	100.52	99.94	10.98
所有部位除外皮肤 **All sites exc.C44**	15 411	226.92	99.43	100.06	99.46	10.95

	女性 Female					
例数 No.cases	粗率 Crude rate (1/10^5)	构成比 Freq.(%)	中标率 ASR China (1/10^5)	世标率 ASR World (1/10^5)	累积率 Cumulative rate (0~74, %)	ICD10
94	1.38	0.89	0.52	0.51	0.05	C00-10, C12-14
18	0.26	0.17	0.11	0.11	0.01	C11
202	2.96	1.92	0.91	0.90	0.07	C15
552	8.10	5.23	3.57	3.41	0.33	C16
1 290	18.92	12.23	6.83	6.74	0.61	C18-21
635	9.31	6.02	3.63	3.58	0.38	C22
394	5.78	3.74	2.21	2.14	0.21	C23-24
554	8.12	5.25	3.12	3.08	0.34	C25
13	0.19	0.12	0.05	0.05	0.00	C32
2 540	37.25	24.08	14.16	13.84	1.42	C33-34
49	0.72	0.46	0.34	0.33	0.04	C37-38
49	0.72	0.46	0.40	0.37	0.04	C40-41
26	0.38	0.25	0.20	0.18	0.02	C43
1 067	15.65	10.12	7.40	7.29	0.81	C50
237	3.48	2.25	2.07	1.92	0.20	C53
240	3.52	2.28	1.61	1.59	0.20	C54-55
473	6.94	4.48	3.44	3.38	0.41	C56
—	—	—	—	—	—	C61
—	—	—	—	—	—	C62
308	4.52	2.92	1.52	1.54	0.12	C64-66, C68
191	2.80	1.81	0.85	0.85	0.06	C67
254	3.73	2.41	2.04	1.98	0.20	C70-C72
71	1.04	0.67	0.45	0.44	0.05	C73
407	5.97	3.86	2.53	2.50	0.28	C81-85, C88, C90, C96
340	4.99	3.22	2.60	2.58	0.26	C91-95, D45-47
543	7.95	5.16	3.27	3.28	0.30	Other
10 547	154.68	100.00	63.83	62.58	6.41	All
10 503	154.03	99.58	63.64	62.38	6.40	All sites exc.C44

附表 3 2017 年北京市城区户籍居民恶性肿瘤发病主要指标

Appendix table 3 Incidence of all cancers in urban areas of Beijing, 2017

部位 Sites	男性 Male					
	例数 No.cases	粗率 Crude rate （1/10^5）	构成比 Freq.（%）	中标率 ASR China （1/10^5）	世标率 ASR World （1/10^5）	累积率 Cumulative rate（0~74,%）
口腔 Oral cavity & pharynx	260	6.18	1.61	3.13	3.17	0.36
鼻咽 Nasopharynx	32	0.76	0.20	0.56	0.49	0.05
食管 Esophagus	519	12.33	3.22	5.34	5.50	0.66
胃 Stomach	1 122	26.65	6.96	11.86	11.72	1.41
结直肠 Colon-rectum	2 519	59.84	15.63	27.47	27.27	3.34
肝脏 Liver	1 021	24.25	6.34	11.60	11.64	1.31
胆囊 Gallbladder etc.	333	7.91	2.07	3.44	3.40	0.40
胰腺 Pancreas	532	12.64	3.30	5.76	5.70	0.70
喉 Larynx	163	3.87	1.01	1.84	1.90	0.23
肺 Lung	3 718	88.32	23.07	38.98	38.91	4.79
其他胸腔器官 Other thoracic organs	52	1.24	0.32	0.75	0.69	0.08
骨 Bone	61	1.45	0.38	1.22	1.15	0.08
皮肤黑色素瘤 Melanoma of skin	24	0.57	0.15	0.29	0.26	0.03
乳腺 Breast	19	0.45	0.12	0.21	0.20	0.02
子宫颈 Cervix	—	—	—	—	—	—
子宫体 Uterus	—	—	—	—	—	—
卵巢 Ovary	—	—	—	—	—	—
前列腺 Prostate	1 187	28.20	7.37	11.94	11.72	1.55
睾丸 Testis	28	0.67	0.17	0.67	0.61	0.05
肾 Kidney	889	21.12	5.52	11.28	10.95	1.31
膀胱 Bladder	865	20.55	5.37	8.85	8.75	1.03
脑 Brain	199	4.73	1.24	3.40	3.34	0.31
甲状腺 Thyroid	818	19.43	5.08	18.74	15.19	1.30
淋巴瘤 Lymphoma	530	12.59	3.29	6.87	6.61	0.74
白血病 Leukemia	452	10.74	2.81	6.44	6.78	0.61
其他 Other	770	18.28	4.77	9.17	9.51	0.93
所有部位合计 All sites	16 113	382.76	100.00	189.81	185.47	21.29
所有部位除外皮肤 　All sites exc.C44	15 940	378.65	98.93	187.85	183.57	21.08

	女性 Female					
例数 No.cases	粗率 Crude rate （1/10⁵）	构成比 Freq.（%）	中标率 ASR China （1/10⁵）	世标率 ASR World （1/10⁵）	累积率 Cumulative rate （0~74，%）	ICD10
174	4.11	1.03	2.04	1.90	0.21	C00-10, C12-14
16	0.38	0.09	0.15	0.15	0.02	C11
140	3.31	0.83	1.05	1.03	0.09	C15
579	13.69	3.43	6.18	5.93	0.66	C16
1 818	42.97	10.77	18.16	17.75	2.06	C18-21
446	10.54	2.64	4.03	4.07	0.43	C22
318	7.52	1.88	2.73	2.68	0.30	C23-24
431	10.19	2.55	3.83	3.78	0.41	C25
12	0.28	0.07	0.10	0.10	0.01	C32
2 730	64.53	16.17	28.29	27.83	3.22	C33-34
37	0.87	0.22	0.47	0.50	0.05	C37-38
34	0.80	0.20	0.52	0.48	0.05	C40-41
32	0.76	0.19	0.51	0.48	0.05	C43
3 468	81.97	20.54	49.50	46.65	5.20	C50
391	9.24	2.32	6.58	5.92	0.59	C53
853	20.16	5.05	11.73	11.44	1.34	C54-55
544	12.86	3.22	7.85	7.49	0.83	C56
—	—	—	—	—	—	C61
—	—	—	—	—	—	C62
556	13.14	3.29	6.03	5.94	0.68	C64-66, C68
331	7.82	1.96	3.07	3.03	0.36	C67
201	4.75	1.19	3.12	3.13	0.28	C70-C72
2 256	53.33	13.36	48.07	40.25	3.63	C73
453	10.71	2.68	5.58	5.32	0.61	C81-85, C88, C90, C96
308	7.28	1.82	4.74	4.86	0.46	C91-95, D45-47
756	17.89	4.50	9.13	9.01	0.92	Other
16 884	399.10	100.00	223.46	209.72	22.46	All
16 733	395.53	99.11	221.10	208.03	22.28	All sites exc.C44

附表 4 2017 年北京市城区户籍居民恶性肿瘤死亡主要指标

Appendix table 4 Mortality of all cancers in urban areas of Beijing, 2017

部位 Sites	男性 Male					
	例数 No.cases	粗率 Crude rate （1/10⁵）	构成比 Freq.（%）	中标率 ASR China （1/10⁵）	世标率 ASR World （1/10⁵）	累积率 Cumulative rate(0~74,%）
口腔 Oral cavity & pharynx	140	3.33	1.40	1.44	1.48	0.18
鼻咽 Nasopharynx	49	1.16	0.49	0.66	0.62	0.07
食管 Esophagus	462	10.97	4.63	4.45	4.58	0.54
胃 Stomach	768	18.24	7.69	7.04	6.91	0.73
结直肠 Colon-rectum	1 219	28.96	12.21	10.89	10.77	1.08
肝脏 Liver	977	23.21	9.79	10.54	10.50	1.16
胆囊 Gallbladder etc.	252	5.99	2.52	2.30	2.30	0.26
胰腺 Pancreas	521	12.38	5.22	5.40	5.36	0.68
喉 Larynx	61	1.45	0.61	0.55	0.55	0.06
肺 Lung	3 013	71.57	30.18	28.03	28.08	3.25
其他胸腔器官 Other thoracic organs	47	1.12	0.47	0.53	0.50	0.06
骨 Bone	34	0.81	0.34	0.56	0.54	0.04
皮肤黑色素瘤 Melanoma of skin	21	0.50	0.21	0.20	0.20	0.01
乳腺 Breast	4	0.10	0.04	0.03	0.03	0.00
子宫颈 Cervix	—	—	—	—	—	—
子宫体 Uterus	—	—	—	—	—	—
卵巢 Ovary	—	—	—	—	—	—
前列腺 Prostate	455	10.81	4.56	3.20	3.15	0.22
睾丸 Testis	6	0.14	0.06	0.10	0.09	0.01
肾 Kidney	321	7.63	3.22	3.01	3.04	0.34
膀胱 Bladder	356	8.46	3.57	2.42	2.51	0.19
脑 Brain	138	3.28	1.38	1.81	1.78	0.18
甲状腺 Thyroid	25	0.59	0.25	0.23	0.23	0.03
淋巴瘤 Lymphoma	341	8.10	3.42	3.33	3.24	0.36
白血病 Leukemia	338	8.03	3.39	3.64	3.63	0.37
其他 Other	434	10.30	4.35	4.19	4.26	0.41
所有部位合计 All sites	9 982	237.12	100.00	94.55	94.35	10.23
所有部位除外皮肤 All sites exc.C44	9 910	235.41	99.28	94.02	93.80	10.19

女性 Female						
例数 No.cases	粗率 Crude rate (1/10^5)	构成比 Freq.（%）	中标率 ASR China (1/10^5)	世标率 ASR World (1/10^5)	累积率 Cumulative rate （0~74，%）	ICD10
63	1.49	0.90	0.52	0.51	0.05	C00-10, C12-14
14	0.33	0.20	0.12	0.12	0.01	C11
128	3.03	1.83	0.80	0.79	0.05	C15
387	9.15	5.53	3.68	3.56	0.35	C16
892	21.08	12.74	6.79	6.76	0.63	C18-21
400	9.46	5.71	3.17	3.16	0.31	C22
238	5.63	3.40	1.90	1.82	0.17	C23-24
396	9.36	5.65	3.26	3.24	0.35	C25
9	0.21	0.13	0.05	0.05	0.00	C32
1 589	37.56	22.69	12.86	12.52	1.27	C33-34
36	0.85	0.51	0.41	0.38	0.04	C37-38
16	0.38	0.23	0.26	0.22	0.02	C40-41
17	0.40	0.24	0.20	0.19	0.02	C43
745	17.61	10.64	7.90	7.82	0.90	C50
140	3.31	2.00	1.94	1.78	0.18	C53
170	4.02	2.43	1.73	1.71	0.21	C54-55
318	7.52	4.54	3.59	3.54	0.43	C56
—	—	—	—	—	—	C61
—	—	—	—	—	—	C62
230	5.44	3.28	1.59	1.59	0.11	C64-66, C68
138	3.26	1.97	0.83	0.82	0.06	C67
158	3.73	2.26	2.05	2.00	0.21	C70-C72
49	1.16	0.70	0.47	0.47	0.05	C73
277	6.55	3.95	2.59	2.53	0.29	C81-85, C88, C90, C96
229	5.41	3.27	2.74	2.75	0.27	C91-95, D45-47
365	8.63	5.20	3.27	3.29	0.33	Other
7 004	165.56	100.00	62.72	61.62	6.31	All
6 978	164.94	99.63	62.56	61.45	6.30	All sites exc.C44

附表 5 2017 年北京市郊区户籍居民恶性肿瘤发病主要指标

Appendix table 5 Incidence of all cancers in peri-urban areas of Beijing, 2017

部位 Sites	男性 Male					
	例数 No.cases	粗率 Crude rate （1/10^5）	构成比 Freq.（%）	中标率 ASR China （1/10^5）	世标率 ASR World （1/10^5）	累积率 Cumulative rate(0~74,%)
口腔 Oral cavity & pharynx	128	4.96	1.48	2.77	2.76	0.32
鼻咽 Nasopharynx	24	0.93	0.28	0.59	0.54	0.06
食管 Esophagus	445	17.24	5.15	8.64	8.77	1.02
胃 Stomach	545	21.11	6.31	11.26	11.18	1.32
结直肠 Colon-rectum	1 101	42.64	12.74	22.66	22.52	2.70
肝脏 Liver	649	25.14	7.51	14.03	14.01	1.63
胆囊 Gallbladder etc.	239	9.26	2.77	4.64	4.61	0.53
胰腺 Pancreas	279	10.81	3.23	5.80	5.66	0.73
喉 Larynx	111	4.30	1.28	2.27	2.25	0.28
肺 Lung	2 323	89.97	26.89	46.57	46.45	5.82
其他胸腔器官 Other thoracic organs	40	1.55	0.46	0.99	0.98	0.12
骨 Bone	42	1.63	0.49	1.55	1.53	0.13
皮肤黑色素瘤 Melanoma of skin	12	0.46	0.14	0.29	0.27	0.03
乳腺 Breast	12	0.46	0.14	0.24	0.23	0.02
子宫颈 Cervix	—	—	—	—	—	—
子宫体 Uterus	—	—	—	—	—	—
卵巢 Ovary	—	—	—	—	—	—
前列腺 Prostate	419	16.23	4.85	8.06	7.97	0.92
睾丸 Testis	11	0.43	0.13	0.44	0.40	0.03
肾 Kidney	383	14.83	4.43	8.70	8.46	1.02
膀胱 Bladder	392	15.18	4.54	7.92	7.89	0.93
脑 Brain	147	5.69	1.70	4.39	4.15	0.39
甲状腺 Thyroid	391	15.14	4.53	13.64	11.33	0.97
淋巴瘤 Lymphoma	284	11.00	3.29	6.72	6.48	0.72
白血病 Leukemia	245	9.49	2.84	6.56	6.78	0.62
其他 Other	417	16.16	4.82	9.53	9.71	1.04
所有部位合计 All sites	8 639	334.61	100.00	188.25	184.92	21.35
所有部位除外皮肤 All sites exc.C44	8 571	331.97	99.21	186.85	183.54	21.19

			女性 Female			
例数 No.cases	粗率 Crude rate （1/10⁵）	构成比 Freq.（%）	中标率 ASR China （1/10⁵）	世标率 ASR World （1/10⁵）	累积率 Cumulative rate （0~74，%）	ICD10
57	2.20	0.68	1.39	1.30	0.14	C00-10, C12-14
8	0.31	0.09	0.18	0.17	0.02	C11
79	3.05	0.94	1.25	1.26	0.12	C15
225	8.69	2.67	4.70	4.45	0.45	C16
816	31.53	9.68	15.66	15.40	1.81	C18-21
248	9.58	2.94	4.76	4.68	0.52	C22
195	7.53	2.31	3.62	3.53	0.43	C23-24
170	6.57	2.02	3.10	3.06	0.35	C25
5	0.19	0.06	0.08	0.08	0.01	C32
1 354	52.31	16.05	25.99	25.63	2.99	C33-34
18	0.70	0.21	0.37	0.39	0.05	C37-38
27	1.04	0.32	0.81	0.80	0.08	C40-41
11	0.43	0.13	0.19	0.19	0.02	C43
1 651	63.79	19.58	40.89	38.10	4.14	C50
261	10.08	3.09	7.51	6.59	0.64	C53
505	19.51	5.99	11.75	11.35	1.26	C54-55
298	11.51	3.53	7.13	6.89	0.74	C56
—	—	—	—	—	—	C61
—	—	—	—	—	—	C62
264	10.20	3.13	5.35	5.35	0.64	C64-66, C68
139	5.37	1.65	2.68	2.64	0.34	C67
119	4.60	1.41	3.08	3.01	0.26	C70-C72
1 207	46.63	14.31	40.07	34.44	3.07	C73
172	6.65	2.04	3.82	3.71	0.39	C81-85, C88, C90, C96
212	8.19	2.51	5.33	5.54	0.52	C91-95, D45-47
393	15.20	4.66	9.02	8.90	0.86	Other
8 434	325.86	100.00	198.72	187.46	19.85	All
8 348	322.54	98.98	196.98	185.79	19.67	All sites exc.C44

附表 6 2017 年北京市郊区户籍居民恶性肿瘤死亡主要指标

Appendix table 6 Mortality of all cancers in peri-urban areas of Beijing, 2017

部位 Sites	男性 Male					
	例数 No.cases	粗率 Crude rate （1/10^5）	构成比 Freq.（%）	中标率 ASR China （1/10^5）	世标率 ASR World （1/10^5）	累积率 Cumulative rate(0~74,%)
口腔 Oral cavity & pharynx	85	3.29	1.54	1.75	1.78	0.21
鼻咽 Nasopharynx	19	0.74	0.34	0.61	0.60	0.06
食管 Esophagus	394	15.26	7.14	7.55	7.61	0.84
胃 Stomach	395	15.30	7.16	7.74	7.57	0.76
结直肠 Colon-rectum	473	18.32	8.57	9.14	9.10	0.96
肝脏 Liver	637	24.67	11.54	13.38	13.42	1.56
胆囊 Gallbladder etc.	200	7.75	3.62	3.84	3.72	0.40
胰腺 Pancreas	245	9.49	4.44	5.04	4.86	0.63
喉 Larynx	52	2.01	0.94	0.99	0.98	0.11
肺 Lung	1 837	71.15	33.29	36.18	35.75	4.24
其他胸腔器官 Other thoracic organs	23	0.89	0.42	0.54	0.52	0.08
骨 Bone	30	1.16	0.54	0.77	0.75	0.07
皮肤黑色素瘤 Melanoma of skin	11	0.43	0.20	0.23	0.23	0.04
乳腺 Breast	6	0.23	0.11	0.11	0.11	0.01
子宫颈 Cervix	—	—	—	—	—	—
子宫体 Uterus	—	—	—	—	—	—
卵巢 Ovary	—	—	—	—	—	—
前列腺 Prostate	158	6.12	2.86	2.77	2.76	0.21
睾丸 Testis	1	0.04	0.02	0.01	0.02	0.00
肾 Kidney	122	4.73	2.21	2.36	2.40	0.23
膀胱 Bladder	168	6.51	3.04	3.04	3.03	0.24
脑 Brain	105	4.07	1.90	2.65	2.55	0.27
甲状腺 Thyroid	14	0.54	0.25	0.27	0.28	0.02
淋巴瘤 Lymphoma	181	7.01	3.28	3.77	3.66	0.41
白血病 Leukemia	189	7.32	3.43	4.65	4.43	0.42
其他 Other	173	6.69	3.17	3.47	3.49	0.41
所有部位合计 All sites	5 518	213.72	100.00	110.87	109.62	12.18
所有部位除外皮肤 All sites exc.C44	5 501	213.07	99.69	110.56	109.28	12.15

	女性 Female					ICD10
例数 No.cases	粗率 Crude rate （1/10⁵）	构成比 Freq.（%）	中标率 ASR China （1/10⁵）	世标率 ASR World （1/10⁵）	累积率 Cumulative rate （0~74，%）	
31	1.20	0.87	0.52	0.52	0.06	C00-10, C12-14
4	0.15	0.11	0.10	0.09	0.01	C11
74	2.86	2.09	1.13	1.13	0.09	C15
165	6.38	4.66	3.37	3.14	0.29	C16
398	15.38	11.23	6.94	6.71	0.59	C18-21
235	9.08	6.63	4.33	4.23	0.49	C22
156	6.03	4.40	2.76	2.73	0.28	C23-24
158	6.10	4.46	2.83	2.75	0.31	C25
4	0.15	0.11	0.05	0.05	0.00	C32
951	36.74	26.84	16.59	16.31	1.68	C33-34
13	0.50	0.37	0.23	0.24	0.03	C37-38
33	1.28	0.93	0.66	0.64	0.08	C40-41
9	0.35	0.25	0.19	0.17	0.02	C43
322	12.44	9.09	6.59	6.39	0.68	C50
97	3.75	2.74	2.29	2.14	0.22	C53
70	2.70	1.98	1.38	1.36	0.18	C54-55
155	5.99	4.37	3.16	3.11	0.37	C56
—	—	—	—	—	—	C61
—	—	—	—	—	—	C62
78	3.01	2.20	1.32	1.34	0.13	C64-66, C68
53	2.05	1.50	0.85	0.85	0.07	C67
96	2.71	2.71	2.06	1.95	0.20	C70-C72
22	0.85	0.62	0.41	0.41	0.05	C73
130	5.02	3.67	2.42	2.43	0.27	C81-85, C88, C90, C96
111	4.29	3.13	2.38	2.31	0.24	C91-95, D45-47
178	6.88	5.04	3.39	3.34	0.26	Other
3 543	136.89	100.00	65.95	64.34	6.60	All
3 525	136.19	99.49	65.68	64.06	6.59	All sites exc.C44

致 谢
Acknowledgement

《2020 北京肿瘤登记年报》编委会对各医疗机构相关工作人员在本年报出版过程中给予的大力协助，尤其是国家癌症中心 / 全国肿瘤登记中心、北京市卫生健康委员会疾病预防控制处和信息中心在数据报送和质控等方面所做出的贡献，表示衷心感谢。

The editorial committee of *Beijing Cancer Registry Annual Report 2020* would like to express their gratitude to all staff of medical institutions who have made a great contribution for the report, especially National Cancer Center & National Central Cancer Registry, Division of Disease Prevention and Control, Information Center of the Beijing Municipal Health Commission, for their contribution on data reporting and quality control.

2017 年北京市报告肿瘤登记资料医疗机构
The medical institutions which submitted cancer case data in Beijing, 2017

辖区 Districts	医疗机构名单 List of medical institutions
北京市 Beijing	北京市疾病预防控制中心 Beijing Center for Diseases Prevention and Control
东城区 Dongcheng	中国医学科学院北京协和医院 Peking Union Medical College Hospital
	首都医科大学附属北京天坛医院 Beijing Tiantan Hospital, Capital Medical University
	北京医院 Beijing Hospital
	首都医科大学附属北京同仁医院 Beijing Tongren Hospital, Capital Medical University
	首都医科大学附属北京妇产医院 Beijing Obstetrics and Gynecology Hospital, Capital Medical University
	北京市普仁医院 Beijing Puren Hospital
	首都医科大学附属北京中医医院 Beijing Hospital of Traditional Chinese Medicine, Capital Medical University
	北京中医药大学东直门医院 Dongzhimen Hospital, Beijing University of Chinese Medicine
	首都医科大学附属北京口腔医院 Beijing Stomatological Hospital, Capital Medical University
	北京市第六医院 Peking University Sixth Hospital
	北京市隆福医院 Beijing Longfu Hospital

续表

辖区 Districts	医疗机构名单 List of medical institutions
	北京同仁堂中医医院 Beijing Tongrentang Hospital of Traditional Chinese Medicine
	北京市和平里医院 Beijing Hepingli Hospital
	北京市东城区第一人民医院 Beijing Dongcheng District First People's Hospital
	北京市东城区第一妇幼保健院 Beijing Dongcheng First Maternal and Child Health Hospital
	北京市鼓楼中医医院 Beijing Gulou Traditional Chinese Medicine Hospital
西城区 Xicheng	北京大学人民医院 Peking University People's Hospital
	北京大学第一医院 Peking University First Hospital
	首都医科大学附属北京友谊医院 Beijing Friendship Hospital, Capital Medical University
	首都医科大学宣武医院 Xuanwu Hospital, Capital Medical University
	首都医科大学附属北京儿童医院 Beijing Children's Hospital, Capital Medical University
	北京积水潭医院 Beijing Jishuitan Hospital
	中国中医科学院广安门医院 Guang'anmen Hospital, China Academy of Chinese Medical Sciences
	首都医科大学附属复兴医院 Fuxing Hospital, Capital Medical University
	北京市健宫医院 Beijing Jiangong Hospital
	北京市肛肠医院 Beijing Rectum Hospital
	北京市西城区展览路医院 Beijing Zhanlanlu Hospital
	北京市西城区广外医院 Guangwai Hospital of Xicheng District, Beijing
	北京市监狱管理局中心医院 Beijing Prison Administration Central Hospital

辖区 Districts	医疗机构名单 List of medical institutions
	北京市回民医院 Beijing Huimin Hospital
	北京市第二医院 The Second Hospital of Beijing
	北京市宣武中医医院 Beijing Xuanwu Traditional Chinese Medical Hospital
	中国医学科学院阜外医院 Fuwai Hospital Chinese Academy of Medical Sciences
	北京市丰盛中医骨伤专科医院 Beijing Fengsheng Special Hospital of Traditional Medical Traumatology and Orthopaedics
	北京新世纪儿童医院 New Century International Children's Hospital
	北京中医药大学附属护国寺中医医院 Huguosi Hospital of Traditional Chinese Medicine of Beijing University of Chinese Medicine
朝阳区 Chaoyang	中国医学科学院肿瘤医院 Cancer Hospital Chinese Academy of Medical Sciences
	中日友好医院 China-Japan Friendship Hospital
	首都医科大学附属北京朝阳医院 Beijing Chao-Yang Hospital, Capital Medical University
	首都医科大学附属北京安贞医院 Beijing Anzhen Hospital, Capital Medical University
	首都医科大学附属北京地坛医院 Beijing Ditan Hospital, Capital Medical University
	煤炭总医院 Beijing Coal General Hospital
	北京华信医院 Beijing Huaxin Hospital
	中国医科大学航空总医院 Aviation General Hospital, China Medical University
	首都儿科研究所附属儿童医院 Children's Hospital, Capital Institute of Pediatrics
	民航总医院 Civil Aviation General Hospital

辖区 Districts	医疗机构名单 List of medical institutions
	北京市垂杨柳医院 Beijing Chui Yang Liu Hospital
	中国中医科学院望京医院 Wangjing Hospital of China Academy of Chinese Medical Sciences
	北京中医药大学第三附属医院 Beijing University of Chinese Medicine Third Affiliated Hospital
	北京和睦家医院 Beijing United Family Hospital
	北京市第一中西医结合医院 Beijing First Integrated Traditional Chinese and Western Medicine Hospital
	北京市朝阳区妇幼保健院 Chaoyang District Maternal and Child Health Care Hospital
	北京五洲妇儿医院 GlobalCare Women and Children's Hospital
	北京市朝阳区双桥医院 Shuangqiao Hospital of Chaoyang District, Beijing
	北京朝阳急诊抢救中心 Beijing Chaoyang Emergency Medical Center
	北京市朝阳区桓兴肿瘤医院 Cancer Hospital of Huanxing ChaoYang District, Beijing
	中国藏学研究中心北京藏医院 Beijng Tibetan Hospital, China Tibetology Research Center
	北京精诚博爱康复医院 Beijing Jingcheng Boai Rehabilitation Hospital
	北京首都国际机场医院 Beijing Capital International Airport Hospital
	北京华府妇儿医院 Huafu Women and Children's Hospital
	北京百子湾和美妇儿医院 HarMoniCare Beijing Women and Children's Hospital
	北京玛丽妇婴医院 Beijing Mary's Hospital for Women and Children
	北京亚运村美中宜和妇儿医院 Amcare Women's and Children's Hospital
	北京优联耳鼻喉医院 Beijing Unicare EENT Hospital

辖区 Districts	医疗机构名单 List of medical institutions
	北京麦瑞骨科医院 Mary's Orthopedic Hospital, Beijing
	北京市红十字会急诊抢救中心 Red Cross Society of China Beijing Branch
	北京市老年病医院 Beijing Geriatrics Hospital
丰台区 Fengtai	首都医科大学附属北京佑安医院 Beijing Youan Hospital, Capital Medical University
	北京瑶医医院 Beijing Yao Medicine Hospital
	国家电网公司北京电力医院 Beijing Electric Power Hospital
	北京京西肿瘤医院 Western Beijing Cancer Hospital
	北京航天总医院 Beijing Aerospace General Hospital
	北京丰台医院 Beijing Fengtai Hospital
	北京中医药大学东方医院 Dongfang Hospital Beijing University of Chinese Medicine
	中国航天科工集团七三一医院 Aerospace 731 Hospital
	北京博爱医院 Beijing Boai Hospital
	北京长峰医院 Beijing Changfeng Hospital
	北京市丰台中西医结合医院 Beijing Fengtai Hospital of Integrated Traditional and Western Medicine
	北京市丰台区南苑医院 Nanyuan Hospital, Fengtai District, Beijing
	北京市丰台区老年人协会莲花池康复医院 Beijing Lianhuachi Rehabilitation Hospital
	北京市丰台区铁营医院 Tieying Hospital of Fengtai District Beijing
	北京丰台英博中西医结合医院 Beijing Fengtai Yingbo Hospital of Integrated Traditional and Western Medicine

辖区 Districts	医疗机构名单 List of medical institutions
	北京博仁医院 Beijing Boren Hospital
	北京丰台华山医院 Beijing Fengtai Huashan Hospital
	北京六一八厂医院 Beijing 618 Factory Hospital
	北京市丰台区妇幼保健计划生育服务中心 Beijing Fengtai Maternal and Child Health and Family Planning Service Center
	北京市木材厂职工医院 Beijing Timber Factory Worker's Hospital
	北京华坛中西医结合医院 Beijing Huatan Integrative Medicine Hospital
	北京市丰台区妇幼保健院 Fengtai Maternal and Child Health Hospital
	北京市红十字会和平医院 Beijing Red Cross Heping Hospital
石景山区 Shijingshan	北京大学首钢医院 Peking University Shougang Hospital
	北京市石景山医院 Beijing Shijingshan Hospital
	清华大学玉泉医院 Yuquan Hospital Affiliated to Tsinghua University
	首都医科大学附属北京康复医院 Beijing Rehabilitation Hospital of Capital Medical University
	中国中医科学院眼科医院 Eye Hospital China Academy of Chinese Medical Sciences
	中国医学科学院整形外科医院 Plastic Surgery Hospital of Chinese Academy of Medical Sciences
	北京联科中医肾病医院 Beijing United-Tech Nephrology Specialist Hospital
海淀区 Haidian	北京肿瘤医院 Beijing Cancer Hospital
	北京大学第三医院 Peking University Third Hospital
	首都医科大学附属北京世纪坛医院 Beijing Shijitan Hospital, Capital Medical University

辖区 Districts	医疗机构名单 List of medical institutions
	航天中心医院 Aerospace Center Hospital
	首都医科大学三博脑科医院 Sanbo Brain Hospital, Capital Medical University
	北京大学口腔医院 Peking University Hospital of Stomatology
	北京市海淀医院 Beijing Haidian Hospital
	中国中医科学院西苑医院 Xiyuan Hospital China Academy of Chinese Medical Sciences
	北京市中关村医院 Beijing Zhongguancun Hospital
	北京老年医院 Beijing Geriatric Hospital
	北京市海淀区妇幼保健院 Haidian Maternal and Child Health Hospital
	北京水利医院 Beijing Water Conservancy Hospital
	北京市中西医结合医院 Beijing Hospital of Integrated Traditional Chinese and Western Medicine
	北京裕和中西医结合康复医院 Beijing Yuho Rehabilitation Hospital
	北京四季青医院 Beijing Sijiqing Hospital
	清华大学医院 Tsinghua University Hospital
	北京大学医院 Peking University Hospital
	北京德尔康尼骨科医院 Beijing Diakonie Orthopaedic Hospital
门头沟区 Mentougou	北京京煤集团总医院 Beijing Jingmei Group General Hospital
	北京市门头沟区医院 Beijing Mentougou District Hospital
	北京市门头沟区妇幼保健院 Mentougou Maternal and Child Health Hospital

续表

辖区 Districts	医疗机构名单 List of medical institutions
	北京市门头沟区中医医院 Beijing Mentougou Hospital of Traditional Chinese Medicine
房山区 Fangshan	北京市房山区第一医院 The First Hospital of Fangshan District, Beijing
	北京市房山区良乡医院 Liangxiang Hospital, Fangshan District, Beijing
	北京燕化医院 Beijing Yanhua Hospital
	北京市房山区中医医院 Fangshan District Hospital of Traditional Chinese Medicine of Beijing
	北京市房山区妇幼保健院 Fangshan District Maternal and Child Health Hospital
	中国核工业北京四〇一医院 Beijing 401 Hospital, China Nuclear Industry
	北京同济东方中西医结合医院 Beijing Tongji Oriental Hospital of Integrated Traditional and Western Medicine
通州区 Tongzhou	首都医科大学附属北京胸科医院 Beijing Chest Hospital, Capital Medical University
	首都医科大学附属北京潞河医院 Beijing Luhe Hospital, Capital Medical University
	北京市通州区中医医院 Tongzhou Traditional Chinese Medicine Hospital
	北京市通州区妇幼保健院 Tongzhou Maternal and Child Health Hospital of Beijing
	北京市通州区中西医结合医院 Tongzhou District Hospital of Integrative medicine of Beijing
顺义区 Shunyi	北京市顺义区医院 The Hospital of Shunyi District Beijing
	北京市顺义区妇幼保健院 Shunyi District maternal and child health hospital, Beijing
	北京市顺义区中医医院 Beijing Shunyi Hospital of Traditional Chinese Medicine
	北京市顺义区空港医院 Beijing Shunyi Airport Hospital
	首都医科大学附属北京地坛医院顺义院区 Beijing Ditan Hospital, Capital Medical University (Shunyi)

辖区 Districts	医疗机构名单 List of medical institutions
昌平区 Changping	北京大学国际医院 Peking University International Hospital
	北京清华长庚医院 Beijing Tsinghua Changgung Hospital
	北京王府中西医结合医院 Beijing Royal Integrative Medicine Hospital
	北京市昌平区医院 Beijing Changping Hospital
	北京市昌平区中医医院 Chinese Medicine Hospital of Beijing Changping District
	北京京都儿童医院 Beijing Jingdu Children's Hospital
	北京市昌平区妇幼保健院 Changping Women and Children Health Care Hospital
	北京市昌平区中西医结合医院 Beijing Changping Hospital of Integrated Chinese and Western Medicine
	北京大卫中医医院 Beijing David Chinese Medicine Hospital
	北京市昌平区南口医院 Nankou Hospital of Changping District of Beijing
	北京小汤山医院 Beijing Xiaotangshan Hospital
	北京市昌平区沙河医院 Shahe Hospital, Changping District, Beijing
大兴区 Daxing	北京南郊肿瘤医院 Beijing Nanjiao Cancer Hospital
	北京市大兴区人民医院 Renmin Hospital of Daxing District, Beijing
	北京市仁和医院 Beijing Renhe Hospital
	中国中医科学院广安门医院南区 Guang'anmen Hospital, China Academy of Chinese Medical Sciences (South)
	北京市大兴区中西医结合医院 Beijing Daxing District Hospital of Integrated Chinese and Western Medicine
	北京市大兴区妇幼保健院 Beijing Daxing Maternal and Child Care Hospital

续表

辖区 Districts	医疗机构名单 List of medical institutions
怀柔区 Huairou	北京怀柔医院 Beijing Huairou Hospital
	北京市怀柔区中医医院 Huairou Hospital of Traditional Chinese Medicine
	北京市怀柔区妇幼保健院 Huairou District Maternal and Child Health Hospital
	北京康益德中西医结合肺科医院 Beijing Kangyide Integrated Traditional Chinese and Western Medicine Pulmonary Hospital
平谷区 Pinggu	北京市平谷区医院 Beijing Pinggu Hospital
	北京市平谷区中医医院 Beijing Pinggu Traditional Chinese Medicine Hospital
	北京市平谷岳协医院 Yuexie Hospital
	北京市平谷区妇幼保健院 Beijing Pinggu District Maternal and Children Health Care Institute
密云区 Miyun	北京市密云区医院 Hospital of Beijing Miyun District
	北京市密云区妇幼保健院 Maternal and Child Care Service Center of Miyun District in Beijing
	北京市密云区中医医院 Miyun District Hospital of Traditional Chinese Medicine
延庆区 Yanqing	北京市延庆区医院 Beijing Yanqing District Hospital
	北京中医医院延庆医院 Yanqing Hospital of Beijing Chinese Medicine Hospital
	北京市延庆区妇幼保健院 Yanqing Maternal and Child Health Care Hospital of Beijing